Health Through Balance

An Introduction to Tibetan Medicine

Health Through Balance

An Introduction To Tibetan Medicine

Dr. Yeshi Donden

Edited and Translated
By Jeffrey Hopkins

Co-translated by Dr. Lobsang Rabgay
And Alan Wallace

MOTILAL BANARSIDASS PUBLISHERS
PRIVATE LIMITED • DELHI

First South Asian Edition Delhi, 1997
First Edition USA, 1986

In Association with
Snow Lion Publications
P.O. Box 6483
Ithaca, NY 14851
USA

ISBN: 81-208-1519-X

Library of Congress Cataloging-in-Publication Data

Yeshi Dönden, 1929-
Health through balance.
Bibliography : p.
Includes index.
1. Medicine, Tibetan.   I. Hopkins, Jeffrey.
II. Title.   [DNLM: 1. Medicine, Oriental Traditional—China. WB
50 JC6 Y42h] R603. T5Y47   1986   610   86-1879
ISBN: 81-208-1519-X

Also available at:

MOTILAL BANARSIDASS

41 U.A. Bungalow Road, Jawahar Nagar, Delhi 110 007
8 Mahalaxmi Chamber, Warden Road, Mumbai 400 026
120 Royapettah High Road, Mylapore, Chennai 600 004
Sanas Plaza, Subhash Nagar, Pune 411 002
16 St. Mark's Road, Bangalore 560 001
8 Camac Street, Calcutta 700 017
Ashok Rajpath, Patna 800 004
Chowk, Varanasi 221 001

PRINTED IN INDIA

BY JAINENDRA PRAKASH JAIN AT SHRI JAINENDRA PRESS,
A-45 NARAINA INDUSTRIAL AREA, PHASE I, NEW DELHI 110 028
AND PUBLISHED BY NARENDRA PRAKASH JAIN FOR
MOTILAL BANARSIDASS PUBLISHERS PRIVATE LIMITED,
BUNGALOW ROAD, DELHI 110 007

Contents

6 *Health Through Balance*

Preface

During the Spring Semester of 1980 Dr. Yeshi Donden, then personal physician to His Holiness the Dalai Lama, gave an introductory course on Tibetan Medicine at the University of Virginia under the auspices of the Center for South Asian Studies. The lectures provide a glimpse into the complicated and esoteric field of Tibetan medicine. The Tibetan system, mainly derived from Indian Buddhist medicine, centers around restoring and maintaining balance between three physical factors — the three humors called wind (air), bile, and phlegm. (Though "bile", for instance, includes the bile secreted by the gall bladder, it is much more, for it is also the fluid responsible for good sight, a strong mental outlook, and so forth. Thus, the meanings of "wind", "bile", and "phlegm" are very wide.) Treatment for restoring and maintaining balance within these easily disturbed factors is through diet, behavior, medicine, and accessory therapy — the basic system having been enhanced with the practical findings of experienced Tibetan physicians who have used the system for more than a thousand years.

Dr. Yeshi Donden, after escaping to India during the Tibetan uprising in 1959, was appointed the personal physician to His Holiness the Dalai Lama, now in exile in northern India. Through treating members of the Indian government, the Indian army, movie stars, and so forth, Dr. Donden has gained wide fame in many parts of India. People travel from Calcutta, Delhi, and Bombay to his small complement of offices on a hillside in Dharmsala to be treated by a doctor whom many, it is clear, regard with great faith based on results that they have experienced. Dr. Donden himself is a jovial, out-going person who has borne well the rigors of re-establishing the Tibetan Medical Center and then developing his own extensive private practice in India.

His lectures begin with the origins of disease — the distant causes being the basic ignorance of beings wandering in cyclic existence due to not understanding the nature of phenomena and consequently being drawn into desire, hatred, and obscuration. These establish mind-patterns which, in turn, bring about imbalances respectively in wind, bile, and phlegm — the imbalances manifesting as myriad diseases. Dr. Donden holistically considers factors of personality, season, age, climatic condition, diet, behavior, and physical surroundings in addressing the means for restoring health.

From my own experience, albeit not that of a medical doctor but as a patient, the great strength of Tibetan medicine is that it is oriented around patients' symptoms and thus is delicately responsive to symptom clusters, no complaint being disregarded. Tibetan medicine no doubt does not have all the answers, but it has a host of techniques to respond to complicated, long-term symptom patterns. My hope is that competent persons will investigate the Tibetan medical system in a truly scientific manner so that the many benefits for chronic diseases such as hepatitis that a number of us travelling and studying in India have confirmed through our own bodies can be communicated to other parts of the world.

We are fortunate that at this time of tremendous advance

in modern medical techniques there is also recognition that no one system has all the answers, and thus many have an openness to naturopathic forms of medical theory and possible cures. It is particularly fortunate that a very ancient form of medicine has remained almost entirely free from modern influence in Tibet and that at this point of the Tibetan diaspora their system can be analyzed, not just as part of medical history but also as a possible source of curative insights.

The first eight chapters as well as the one on virilification were first translated by Ven. Lobsang Rabgay, a Tibetan monk who accompanied Dr. Donden to the U.S. and who has since earned a Ph.D. in medicine in India. The ninth chapter was first translated by Ven. Jhampa Kelsang (B. Alan Wallace), a student of Tibetan Buddhism and Tibetan medicine for fifteen years and translator of Dr. Donden's book *The Ambrosia Heart Tantra*. I originally translated the remaining chapters and then later re-translated and edited the entire text. Because of its free-flowing form of oral lectures, the book provides an accessible introduction to the vast store of Tibetan perspectives on health.

About the author. Dr. Yeshi Donden was born in 1929 to a prosperous farming family in the southern part of central Tibet in the village of Namro in a district called Hlo-ga, one day's ride from Lhasa.[1] At age six, his parents sent him to a small monastery of around four hundred monks, and then at age eleven he was sent to the Medical College of the capital of Tibet, Hla-sa, due to his considerable abilities at memorization. There, he memorized the four Medical Tantras and then entered into formal training under the Director of the College, Kyen-rap-nor-bu.[2] As John Avedon reports in his *New York Times* interview of January 11, 1981:

> When he was 20, Yeshi Donden scored third in his class behind his two roommates. But because the three scores were so close, the young men were retested. Eyes

10 *Health Through Balance*

closed, they were asked to identify the plants on the basis of taste and smell alone. "I was graduating that year," recalled Dr. Donden in his understated way. "My friends made little mistakes so I would come in first."

Dr. Donden began medical practice in 1951, returning to his own district and developing a high reputation for effectiveness. Then, when the Dalai Lama fled from the Chinese Communists in 1959, Dr. Donden also decided to leave Tibet for India, where he began treating Tibetan refugee patients.

With his appointment as the Dalai Lama's personal physician, he moved to Dharamsala, where he also took on the burden of founding a Tibetan Medical Center. Succeeding at that task despite the tremendous difficulties of the refugee situation, he returned to private practice in 1969, seeing a large number of patients from various walks of life and remaining as the Dalai Lama's physician until 1980. Dr. Donden continues to serve a great number of patients daily, in between frequent trips to the West to lecture on and demonstrate Tibetan medicine. His vast experience shines through the series of lectures given at the University of Virginia which comprise this book.

I wish to thank Dr. Barry Clarke for identifying many of the plants, animals, and minerals and making many helpful suggestions.

Jeffrey Hopkins
Charlottesville, Virginia

Technical Note

In the notes, the names of Tibetan authors and orders are given in "essay phonetics" for the sake of easy pronunciation; for a discussion of the system used, see the Technical Note at the beginning of *Meditation on Emptiness*, pp. 19–22. Transliteration of Tibetan in parentheses and in the glossary is done in accordance with a system devised by Turrell Wylie; see "A Standard System of Tibetan Transcription", *Harvard Journal of Asiatic Studies*, Vol. 22, 1959, pp. 261–7. For the names of Indian scholars and systems used in the body of the text, *ch*, *sh*, and *ṣh* are used instead of the more usual *c*, *ś*, and *ṣ* for the sake of easy pronunciation by non-specialists.

INTRODUCTION

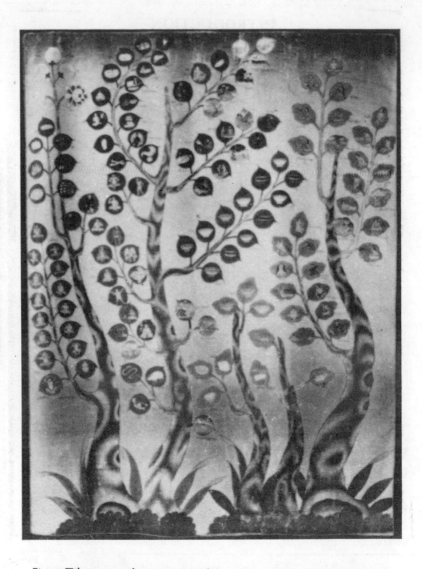

Fig. 1 Tibetan medicine tree with its two major root systems:
a) the body root which supports 2 trunks, 12 branches, 88 leaves, 2 flowers and 3 fruits.
b) the diagnosis root which supports 3 trunks, 8 branches and 38 leaves.

1 Outline of Disease

In this world, all breathing creatures, all beings — whether human beings, animals, whatever — are exposed to different forms of suffering. In the Tibetan system we believe that whether we are physically healthy or not, basically all of us are sick. Even though disease might not be manifest, it is present in dormant form. This fact makes the scope of disease difficult to fathom.

THE ORIGINS OF ILLNESS

With respect to the origins of illness, Shākyamuni Buddha propounded that there are 84,000 different types of afflictive emotions, such as desire and hatred, which have corresponding effects on beings, thus producing 84,000 different types of disorders. These can be condensed into 1,016 types of disorders which can further be condensed into 404.

The factors giving rise to disorders are causes and conditions, the latter enabling the causes to ripen or manifest. Causes are of two different types — distant and proximate. The proximate causes are wind, bile, and phlegm.[3] With regard to the distant ones, the distinct causes for each disorder are difficult to enumerate because basically all disorders have their origin in the mental environment of the past — prior afflictive emotions — and it is these mental factors that are ultimately responsible for all types of disorders. These afflictive emotions impel actions (*karma*) that establish potencies in the mind, ripening later as specific diseases. Hence, it is impossible to determine all the *specific* distant causes involved in a particular disease; however, the *basic* entities of those causes are the afflictive emotions of desire, hatred, and obscuration. These three, in turn, depend upon ignorance.

Ignorance refers to a state of mind that not only is not aware of how things actually exist, but also misconceives the nature of phenomena. Ignorance gives rise to desire which, in turn, leads to hatred, pride, jealousy, harsh speech, more obscuration, and so forth. In rough terms, from the activity of these negative states of mind arise the three types of humoral disorders of wind, bile, and phlegm. Forty-two types of wind disorders arise in dependence upon desire; twenty-six types of bile disorders arise in dependence upon factors of hatred such as pride and jealousy, and thirty-three types of phlegm disorders arise in dependence upon obscuration — making a total of one hundred and one diseases.

CLASSIFICATION OF DISEASE

Disorders can be classified by different methods in terms of location in the body, type, environmental factors, and so forth. Here, by considering four classes of these one hundred and one diseases, there come to be four hundred and four:

1 101 disorders that are under the strong influence of actions (*karma*) in previous lifetimes
2 101 disorders of this lifetime — which have their causes in an early period of the life and manifest later in this same lifetime
3 101 disorders involving spirits
4 101 superficial disorders, so called because by simply following proper diet and behavior patterns one can cor-

rect them without having to resort to medication and accessory therapy.

The last type, superficial disorders, may result from improper intake of food — imbalanced diet — or behavior patterns; thus, these are self-curing without resorting to any form of treatment if the temporary conditions of diet and behavior giving rise to them are corrected. However, disorders of one lifetime, which have their cause in an earlier part of your life and manifest at a later time and are related with karma, will usually prove to be fatal unless treated. Seeking treatment is vital in this type of disorder. Moreover, in some cases mere material medication may not suffice; you will have to resort to spiritual practices such as disclosing past ill-deeds (confession), lessening their force by engaging in virtuous practice, and developing an intention to refrain from such deeds in the future. In these cases, virtuous activity and medication work together.

With respect to diseases that involve interference by spirits, there are, according to the Buddhist explanation, unseen forces that can harm an individual, and thus, even if there may not be any visible cause for a disorder, the person can be afflicted with pain and different forms of disorders due to the influence of such spirits. Though treated for a long period of time with medicine, the person does not respond to treatment and continues to suffer. The reason for this is the spirit behind the disease, and unless it is subdued by spiritual methods, no form of therapy — external or otherwise — will be able to free the person from that disorder. When the spirit is exorcised, however, the disease is cured.

With regard to the one hundred and one types of disorders that are due to past actions, Buddhists believe in rebirth, that is, we believe that there are past lives; these types of disorders are attributed to negative actions committed in past lives. When that karma ripens and a disease manifests in the present lifetime, it is very powerful and thus is generally fatal. In Tibet, people with this type of disorder would often renounce all worldly activities and engage in spiritual practices; however, few survive this type of disorder because the disease is a ripening of a powerful action that has been committed in the past.

THE BASIC MEDICAL LITERATURE

The medical teachings of the Buddha are primarily four texts called the Four Tantras.[4] The first is known as the *Root Tantra*.[5] It is a very short text and mainly presents an outline of the whole medical teaching. The second is the *Explanatory Tantra*.[6] It deals with formation of the human body (embryology), anatomy, signs of death, how conditions cause the manifestation of disorders, the characteristics of particular disorders, the functions of wind, bile, and phlegm when these operate properly and how they bring about diseases when imbalanced, and the corresponding medicines required to correct particular disorders. This second tantra also prescribes the diet and behavior patterns for maintaining health and for combatting disorders — for instance, the types of food one should refrain from, the quality and quantity of food that one should take, and different types of behavior — seasonal behavior, daily behavior, and temporary behavior.

The third, the *Oral Tradition Tantra*,[7] is an extensive technical textbook that identifies the different types of disorders — their causation (etiology), nature (pathology), and therapy. It presents each of the major disorders individually and in great detail — discussing their causes, conditions, and symptoms as well as the methods of treatment to be used.

The fourth, called the *Last Tantra*,[8] deals with methods of diagnosis such as urinalysis and pulse-taking as well as the manufacture of medicines.

CHRONIC DISORDERS

In particular, in the third text, the *Oral Tradition Tantra*, it is explained that this is a period of ruination, beings having coarse behavior, pride, desire, hatred, and obscuration — householders having no ethics and clergy not being without lust. Buddha mentioned that later during this period of degeneration, human beings would develop various types of chemicals that would lead to different types of disorders, called the eighteen malignant or critical disorders during the era of degeneration.

Types of cancer and so forth that are prevalent nowadays but were not so in the past are found among these eighteen types of critical, malignant disorders. These can be further classified in terms of wind, bile, and phlegm and combinations of these, each having eighteen types with individual subdivisions.

We can also categorize types of cancer, for instance, by referring to the four classifications outlined earlier. In those terms, there are tumors having superficial factors involved — caused by improper diet and behavior patterns; these are naturally curable by restoring good diet and behavior patterns. Then, there are types caused by factors within one lifetime which if treated can be cured but, if untreated, can prove fatal. Those caused by spirits are very difficult to treat and will generally prove fatal unless spiritual methods are employed. Then, there are cancers that have their origin in a negative action committed in a previous lifetime; this final type of cancer cannot be cured by any physician.

Another way in which these critical disorders are further classified is in terms of the area or location affected — the vital organs, reservoir organs, vessels, bone, flesh, the sense organs, and so forth. Tumors, also, are described separately from these eighteen critical disorders under a classification of eleven types — these being related with the five vital organs (heart, lungs, liver, spleen, and kidneys) and the six reservoir organs (stomach, small intestine, large intestine, gall bladder, seminal vesicle, and urinary bladder). Again, these are further treated in terms of tumors on the surface, inside, and inbetween; for instance, on the surface, inside, or inbetween the surface and the inner part of a lung, liver, or the stomach.

From my own experience I have found Tibetan medicine to be effective in certain cases of cancer. Several Indian patients who were considered terminal cases have been greatly helped by Tibetan medication over the past several years; some report this in person, others have written to this effect. I will not make claims that there have been a great many.

Other types of disorders for which I have found Tibetan medicine to be extremely effective are hepatitis, certain types of mental disorders, ulcers, paralysis, gallstones, kidney stones, and arthritis. Thus, from my own practice I have found that our system of medicine has proved to be effective for several chronic disorders.

This has been a general introduction or outline of the types of illness; they are described in great detail in the texts.

2 Course of Study

How is Tibetan medicine studied? As mentioned earlier, there are four primary medical texts which Tibetan medical students have to study. During a year or two of preliminary study, they have to memorize at least three of the Four Tantras, these being the first, second, and fourth — *Root Tantra*, *Explanatory Tantra*, and *Last Tantra*. The third, the *Oral Tradition Tantra*, need only be studied, not necessarily memorized during this preliminary time.

Then, during the first year of actual study, medical students study the *Root Tantra* with the help of visual aids called the "Illustrated Trees of Medicine." Three trees are used to illustrate physiology and causation, diagnosis, and treatment. During the second year they study the *Explanatory Tantra*, beginning with embryology and emphasizing causation. In the third year they study the *Last Tantra* which deals with diagnosis, particularly methods of urinalysis and pulse taking, two of the most important forms of diagnosis a Tibetan doctor uses in determining a patient's disorder. After that, during the fourth year, or even longer periods, they spend time in a clinic with a doctor, observing how all the topics learned are applied in practice; they also study medical commentaries.

In Tibetan medicine, physicians and pharmacologists are not separate persons. A doctor must know all aspects of medicine. Therefore, especially during the summer, students accompany physicians to the mountains to study herbs and plants, taking particular notice of their potencies, faults, and advantageous qualities. Then during the winter, they learn how to manufacture medicines. Thereby, they learn all aspects of medical practice.

Regarding the people who trained in Tibetan medicine before the Communist Chinese takeover, most doctors were monks. However, each district in the country selected two lay candidates and sent them to attend the Medical and Astrological College in Hla-sa, the capital of Tibet — one to become a doctor and one to become an astrologer. Apart from these two candidates from each district, two monks were selected from each of the major monasteries to attend the medical college. Thus, there were two categories of selections — lay students selected by district authorities and monks from major monastic centers.

On completion of medical school, lay students returned to their district to practice. Of the monk students, one had to stay at the medical school to engage in practice or research there, and the other had to return to his monastery to practice.

ORIGIN OF THE FOUR MEDICAL TANTRAS

Regarding how the basic four medical texts originated, during an earlier time the Medicine Buddha appeared in this world, displayed the twelve deeds of a Buddha, including becoming enlightened and teaching trainees. He prophesied that in the future the fourth Buddha, Shākyamuni Buddha, would manifest as the Medicine Buddha in India for the sake of trainees.

Later, when Shākyamuni Buddha manifested as the Medicine Buddha, from his heart was manifested Akṣhobhya; from the crown, Vairochana; from the throat, Amitābha who requested the teaching; from the navel, Ratnasambhava; and from the secret region, Amoghasiddhi. Akṣhobhya, Vairochana, Ratnasambhava, and Amoghasiddhi taught the four medical tantras; however, it actually was the Medicine Buddha in the form of the Buddhas of these four lineages who revealed the teachings.

The *Root Tantra* was taught by Akṣhobhya; the *Explanatory Tantra*, by Vairochana; the *Oral Tradition Tantra*, by Ratnasambhava; and the *Last Tantra*, by Amoghasiddhi. Amitābha, entity of the wisdom of individual investigation, requested each teaching. Thus, the Medicine Buddha first emanated Amitābha, who requested the Medicine Buddha for the teaching. This request was accepted, and each of the other four Buddhas were emanated, thereupon giving their respective teachings. As in the *Guhyasamāja Tantra*, the speakers and requester are all the same being.

CONTENTS OF THE FOUR TANTRAS

The *Root Tantra* consists of six sections, the initial major topic being the healthy body.[9] This is called the ordinary untransformed body, meaning that the three humors — wind, bile, and phlegm — are not acting as direct causes of disorders. Nevertheless, disease is naturally present in dormant form; the conditions to cause it to manifest have not yet been encountered. The three humors are, therefore, in a state of balance, not imbalanced.

It is important to remember that the three humors exist in all beings, acting as factors maintaining good health when they are not imbalanced and acting as causes of disease the moment they become imbalanced. Thus, their function is dual; in the state of balance they perform the functions of a healthy body, helping to keep good health, but the moment they are disturbed, these very three turn into causes of physical and mental disorders.

In this section on the healthy body, the *Root Tantra* mainly treats these three types of humors, with five varieties each, as well as the functions of all fifteen — the most important topic in Tibetan medicine. It also explains the activities of the five winds, five biles, and five phlegms when, in a state of imbalance, they promote disease. The *Root Tantra* also briefly speaks about symptoms of disorders and methods of healing as well as mentioning in a brief way topics that are discussed in detail in the other three tantras.

The first seven chapters of the second text, the *Explanatory Tantra*, deal with the formation of the embryo, development of the fetus, birth, and so on right through to death. They also discuss how the five winds, biles, and phlegms function when in balance to maintain health in the body — how they function *individually* as well as the *general* qualities of wind, bile, and phlegm. These seven chapters finish with the process and signs of death, either due to disease or otherwise.

The next three chapters deal with the causes, conditions, and classifications of diseases. Conditions are those factors that help the cause to manifest as a particular disease. This means that even if the cause is present, if the conditions are not, the disease will not manifest. Then, it details the classifications of diseases, at the end of which it describes the characteristics of types of disease.

The following chapters describe the tastes of medicinal ingredients, their potencies, and post-digestive effects. The tastes of medicinal ingredients are important as indicators of their potencies with respect to counteracting disorders. After speaking of the potencies of ingredients in terms of their tastes, these chapters detail how medications with different tastes and potencies work. Finally, they speak of the post-digestive potencies of drugs — how they work after digestion. The action of drugs is slightly different before digestion during the period of ingestion, and then after digestion, when they have been assimilated.

After this, there is discussion of treatment in terms of diet and behavior patterns, these being vital for maintaining good health as well as increasing life span. Diet is treated in terms of the way food should be taken and its quantity as well as recognizing improper diet. Next are chapters on behavior patterns — daily, temporary (such as during the seasons), and continual.

Then there is a section on methods of prolonging life — how to maintain good health by keeping the humors in balance and thus avoiding disease. There is also a section about the methods used to cure different types of disorders, and finally the last section is on the code that physicians should follow in conducting their profession. It talks about commitments, how doctors should regard patients, and so forth. In total, the *Explanatory Tantra* has thirty chapters.

The third text, the *Oral Tradition Tantra*, consists of fifteen main sections with ninety-two chapters in total. These deal with the one hundred and one humoral disorders of wind, bile, and phlegm — the causes and conditions of each of these disorders, the symptoms, therapy consisting of diet and behavior patterns to be recommended for the disorder, and medication to be prescribed once the diet and behavior patterns fail to bring about the requisite cure. Finally, it discusses accessory therapies used if medications fail.

The *Last Tantra* consists of four sections which altogether have twenty-five chapters. The first section deals with diagnosis, the first two chapters of which describe urinalysis and pulse reading. The second section deals with the preparation of medicines — their content, nature, potencies, and so forth — in the form of pills, powdered medicine, syrups, desiccated medication, medicinal butters, and so forth. After that, the third section discusses pacifying, or alleviative, medications — purgatives and emetics — and then, those types of medication that actually destroy or completely subdue disorders. Last is a section dealing with accessory therapy in mild and severe forms, used if the initial herbal medication fails to bring about the cure and also as a preventive form of medication. These include moxa, acupuncture, surgery, and so forth.

That is an outline of the contents of the four primary

medical textbooks. Later, I will discuss relevant sections and chapters in some detail.

BASIC CAUSE OF DISEASE

What is the essential point of these many topics? The most important point concerns ignorance, for the entities and causes of all illness derive from ignorance. From ignorance, there is obscuration, due to which we do not recognize unsalutary states of mind as faulty and instead generate desire that leads to many ill-deeds and the accumulation of bad karma. Similarly, obscuration leads to hatred, resulting in, for instance, the speaking of harsh words, insults, and attacking others. Likewise, jealousy generates senseless competitiveness, and pride causes one to look down on others.

In brief, the three basic afflictive emotions, called the three poisons, are desire, hatred, and obscuration. From obscuration, which is heavy, dull, and cloudy, phlegm disorders increase, phlegm being heavy and viscous. From desire, which has a nature of captivation of the mind, all types of wind disorders arise — wind having a nature of being light and moving. Due to this correspondence, desire produces wind disorders. Hatred is like fire; from it, bile disorders as well as blood-bile disorders arise.

The root is beginningless ignorance. Due to its force we are caught in cyclic existence, in the round of repeated birth, aging, sickness, and death. Ignorance is with us like our own shadow; thus, even if we think that there is no reason to be ill, even if we think that we are in very good health, actually we have had the basic cause of illness since beginningless time.

PART ONE

THE BODY

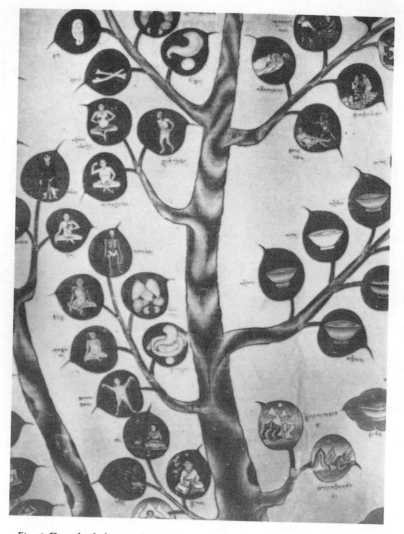

Fig. 2 Detail of the medicine tree which focuses on leaves from the diseased body trunk.

BODY ROOT

2 Trunks, 12 Branches, 88 Leaves, 2 Flowers, 3 Fruits

HEALTHY BODY TRUNK
(1) *Humors Branch*
1. Life-Sustaining Wind
2. Ascending Wind
3. Pervasive Wind
4. Fire-Accompanying Wind
5. Downwards-Voiding Wind
6. Digestive Bile
7. Color-Regulating Bile
8. Determining Bile
9. Sight Bile
10. Complexion-Clearing Bile
11. Supportive Phlegm
12. Decomposing Phlegm
13. Experiencing Phlegm
14. Satisfying Phlegm
15. Connective Phlegm

(2) *Physical Constituents Branch*
1. Nutritional Essence
2. Blood
3. Flesh
4. Fat
5. Bone
6. Marrow
7. Regenerative Fluid

(3) *Excretions Branch*
1. Feces
2. Urine
3. Perspiration

Two Flowers
1. Freedom From Disease
2. Long life

Three Fruits
1. Religious Practice
2. Wealth
3. Happiness

DISEASED BODY TRUNK

(1) *Cause Branch*
    1. Desire (peacock)
    2. Hatred (snake)
    3. Obscuration (pig)

(2) *Condition Branch*
    1. Time/Season
    2. Spirits
    3. Diet
    4. Behavior

(3) *Entrance Branch*
    1. Skin
    2. Flesh
    3. Channels
    4. Bone
    5. Vital Organs (Solid Organs)
    6. Reservoir Organs (Hollow Organs)

(4) *Location Branch*
    1. Brain (Upper Body)
    2. Diaphragm (Middle Body)
    3. Hips, Base of the Spine (Lower Body)

(5) *Pathways Branch*
    Wind Disorders
    1. Bone

2. Ear
3. Skin
4. Heart, Life Channel
5. Large Intestine
Bile Disorders
6. Blood
7. Perspiration
8. Eye
9. Liver
10. Gall Bladder and Small Intestine
Phlegm Disorders
11. Nutritional Essence
12. Stool, Urine
13. Lung, Spleen, and Kidneys
14. Stomach, Urinary Bladder
15. Nose, Tongue

(6) *Time of Arising Branch*
1. Old age
2. Adult
3. Child
4. Cold (wind)
5. Dry (heat)
6. Humid
7. Summer (rainy season)
8. Autumn
9. Spring

(7) *Fatal Effect Branch*
1. Exhaustion of life span, karma, merit
2. Disorder increasing regardless of medication
3. Non-effectiveness of diet, behavior, medicine, accessory therapy
4. Wound in vital organ
5. Severance of continuum of wind in central channel
6. Untreatable heat disorder
7. Untreatable cold disorder

8. Physical constituents cannot accept the medicine
9. Life force stolen by spirits

(8) *Side Effects Branch*
1. Bile arising from wind alleviation
2. Phlegm arising from wind alleviation
3. Bile arising from unsuccessful treatment of wind
4. Phlegm arising from unsuccessful treatment of wind
5. Wind arising from bile alleviation
6. Phlegm arising from bile alleviation
7. Wind arising from unsuccessful treatment of wind
8. Phlegm arising from unsuccessful treatment of wind
9. Wind arising from phlegm alleviation
10. Bile arising from phlegm alleviation
11. Wind arising from unsuccessful treatment of phlegm
12. Bile arising from unsuccessful treatment of phlegm

(9) *Condensation Branch*
1. Cold (wind, phlegm)
2. Hot (blood, bile)

3 Defining the Body

Earlier it was mentioned that the Four Tantras that are the basic textbooks of Tibetan medicine are studied with the help of visual aids in the form of trees, called the "Illustrated Trees of Medicine".[10] There are three roots from which grow nine trunks on which there are forty-two branches; these have 224 leaves, and there are two flowers and three fruits.

The first of the three roots is called "definition of the body".[11] This divides into two trunks, the first being called the trunk of the healthy body abiding in a normal, balanced state and the second, the trunk of the unhealthy body, or diseased body, abiding in an imbalanced state.[12]

Usually, the trees are taught by explaining all three roots together, followed by all nine trunks, then all forty-two branches, then the 224 leaves, and finally the two flowers and three fruits. However, to facilitate understanding, I will explain each root with its respective trunks, branches, and leaves, first briefly and then in more detail. This way you will be able more easily to understand the basic principles of Tibetan medicine.

HEALTHY BODY

(See chart on the preceding pages). The first root, definition of the body, has two trunks — healthy body trunk and unhealthy body trunk. The healthy body trunk has three branches — humors, physical constituents, and excretions.

Humors

The humor branch of the healthy body trunk has three leaves — wind, bile, and phlegm. In the healthy body the three humors of wind, bile, and phlegm are in balance and thus are not promoters of disease as such. For, when they are in a state of balance, the three humors are causes maintaining and improving good health. The moment that they are disturbed, they become causes for disorders; however, as a branch of the healthy body trunk, they are in a state of balance.

Wind is of five types: life-sustaining wind, ascending wind, pervasive wind (existing in all parts of the body), fire-accompanying (or digestive) wind, and downwards-voiding wind.[13] These are the five major types of winds, or currents, that exist in the body.

Similarly, bile is of five types: digestive bile, color or complexion regulating bile, determining bile, sight bile (which enables one to see), and complexion-clearing bile.

Phlegm is also of five types: supportive phlegm, decomposing phlegm, experiencing phlegm (that which experiences tastes), satisfying phlegm, and connective phlegm.

These fifteen types of humors are present in every being; they are factors that carry out the functioning of the body — sustaining the body and enabling it to function in different ways as required. Though basically each being, by the mere fact of having ignorance, is sick, there is no manifest sickness when these fifteen are in balance. When imbalanced, some will have increased and some decreased, resulting in manifest illness. These humors are the fifteen leaves of the humoral branch on the healthy body trunk.

Physical Constituents

The next branch on the healthy body trunk is called the physical constituents, having as leaves the seven types of physical bases that constitute the body: nutritional essence blood, flesh, fat, bone, marrow, and regenerative fluid. Each produces the one after it. Roughly speaking, food that is ingested is separated into refined and unrefined portions, the refined portion being the nutritional essence. It proceeds to the liver where it is made into blood. Blood, in turn, produces flesh, which produces fat, which produces bone, which produces marrow, which produces regenerative fluid. There are many separations into refined and unrefined portions over the course of complete digestion of nutrition.

Excretions

The third branch of the healthy body trunk, the excretion branch, has three leaves: feces, urine, and perspiration. The text explains in detail how these are produced.

Thus, twenty-five leaves grow from the first trunk — fifteen leaves on the humor branch, seven leaves on the physical constituents branch, and the three leaves on the excretion branch. Each requires extensive explanation; right now, I am just identifying the names.

When the body is without disease and long-lived, it is possible to have the three fruits of good health — successful religious practice, wealth, and happiness. In this way, the two flowers of being free from illness and having a long-life ripen into these three fruits.

UNHEALTHY BODY

The second trunk growing from the body root is the diseased body. It has nine branches. The first is the cause branch. The second is the condition branch, conditions being factors which help the cause to ripen, or manifest, as a disease.

The third is the entrance branch — stages through which a disease develops and spreads in various parts of the body once the conditions effect the ripening of the cause. Having entered the body through these various entrances, the disorder then localizes itself in specific areas; thus, the fourth branch is the locations or sites where a disease, after it has entered the body, settles. Here the sites where diseases of predominant wind, bile, or phlegm are localized are described in detail.

The fifth branch is the pathways through which diseases of wind, bile, and phlegm spread in terms of the seven physical constituents and organs mentioned earlier. Having localized in a particular area, a disease spreads through these pathways.

The sixth branch is the time of arising. This refers to how certain factors of age, season, time of the day, and locality promote specific humoral disorders.

The seventh is the fatal effect or result branch; it refers to nine categories of incurable, terminal situations. The eighth branch is side effects resulting from treatment. For instance, as a side effect of treating a wind disorder, a bile disorder could be produced, or from treating a bile disorder a wind disorder could be promoted.

Finally, the ninth branch is a condensation — how ultimately all diseases can be condensed into two categories, cold and hot disorders.

These are the principal topics of Tibetan medicine concerning the etiology, or causation, of disease. Let us now enumerate the leaves on each of the nine branches of the unhealthy body trunk.

Causes
Of the nine branches on the unhealthy body trunk, the first is the cause branch. It has three leaves: desire, hatred, and obscuration which produce wind, bile, and phlegm disorders respectively.

Basically every being on this planet, that is, humans as well as animals, want happiness and do not want any form of disease or suffering. Yet, we do not know how to achieve the causes of happiness and do not know how to get rid of the causes of suffering. According to our own estimation we make great effort at techniques for achieving happiness and avoiding pain, but, instead, mostly generate just the opposite of what we seek — bringing on ourselves more pain and suffering and diminishing whatever happiness we have.

Behind all of this is the powerful force of our former actions, impelled by afflictive emotions — desire, hatred, and ignorance. Thus, when we inquire about the source of disease, we find that there is a force, hidden to our sight that cannot be removed through external medicine or injections — karma, our own former actions and the predispositions they leave in the mind. The root of unfavorable karma, in turn, is the three mental poisons of desire, hatred, and ignorance. The root of all disease is, therefore, these same afflictive emotions of desire, hatred, and ignorance.

If you become able to oppose these afflictive emotions, disease will lessen, you will be more peaceful — everything will be more relaxed. For instance, many people have mentioned how happy most Tibetans are despite the extremely difficult circumstances of being separated from their own country, losing family members, and so forth. This is due to mental attitude.

It is worthwhile to analyze the cause of disease — how disease comes about. We need to understand how, as I mentioned before, ignorance about the status of persons and other phenomena leads us, as if by the nose, into desire and then, stage by stage, into hatred, pride, jealousy, harsh speech, and so on. These are the sources of disease.

It is said that in dependence upon desire, wind disorders are generated. How is this? Being, first of all, under the influence of ignorance, as if led by a ring in the nose, one produces desire, wanting this and wanting that, needing this and needing that. Now, there is no way of achieving *all* of these desires, and most cannot be achieved immediately. When a male or female desires someone else as a partner, this cannot be accomplished merely according to their wish since it also depends upon the other person's wish. Also, even with respect to things, we often do not have the capacity to acquire them. We engage in techniques to get what we want, but often cannot succeed; not achieving what we want, we think too much about these things internally, thereby disturbing the mind. This induces all wind disorders. Desire, therefore, is what leads to wind diseases.

Similarly, hatred increases bile. Out of pride we often overassert ourselves, increasing blood and bile. Through such actions of hatred, which has a nature of being overheated, bile disorders, which also have a nature of heat, are produced.

Again, in dependence upon obscuration, phlegm disorders are created. Obscuration is a case of not knowing one's own faults, of not knowing what is permissible to do and what is not permissible to do; this bewilderment leads us into all sorts of unsuitable actions. Obscuration, involving a heaviness of mind, draws out the corresponding humoral illnesses of phlegm.

Conditions
The second branch on the unhealthy body trunk is the condition branch, which has four leaves. The first is time, such as seasonal factors that allow the causes — wind, bile, and phlegm — to ripen into disorders. If one follows diet or behavior patterns contrary to those recommended for a particular season — for instance, eating too much or too little or wearing too much clothing in summer or too little in winter — a disorder could result. Also, if during a particular season one takes too much or too little medication to account for changes of weather or wrong medication in terms of the season, that could serve as a factor maturing or ripening the causes that one already has. The texts detail diet, behavior patterns, and medications for each season.

The next leaf on the condition branch is spirits that suddenly affect the three humors such that they ripen in the form of a disorder. They are called sudden because these spirits, of which there are many varieties, are encountered when just going from one place to another, for instance. Since they cannot be seen with the eye, they are very difficult to diagnose.

The third leaf is improper diet. When you fail to use discretion regarding the type of diet that your body needs, improper diet can act as a condition causing a disorder to appear. For instance, if after staying in the sun and drinking liquor you take food producing great warmth, such as beef or lamb, a disorder could result.

The fourth and last leaf on the condition branch is improper behavior patterns. For example, if a person wears fur clothing in summer when it is particularly hot, this can act as a condition producing a disorder.

Entrances
The entrance branch refers to the areas through which disorders enter the physical system, once the presence of conditioning factors activates the causes; it has six leaves. First, the disorder resides and spreads in the skin, then develops in the flesh, runs or moves through the channels in the body, adheres to the bone, and descends into the vital organs or the reservoir organs. These are the six stages in the sequence of a disorder once conditions have aggravated the humors, but the sequence may not always occur in every type of disorder.

Locations
The location or site branch has three leaves: upper, middle, and lower parts of the body, called brain, diaphragm, and hips. The upper part refers to the region of the head where phlegm is predominantly located; the middle part, to the upper abdomen where bile is predominantly located; the lower part, to the pelvic region where wind is predominant-

ly located.

Pathways
Next is the pathways branch, which has fifteen leaves, concerned with where diseases of the three humors course in terms of five factors — the seven physical constituents, the five sense organs, the three excretions, the five vital organs, and the six reservoir organs. The predominant pathways where wind disorders course are (1) bone in terms of the physical constituents, (2) ears in terms of the sensory organs, (3) perspiration in terms of the excretions, (4) heart in terms of the vital organs, and (5) large and small intestines in terms of the reservoir organs.

Bile disorders course particularly in (1) the blood in terms of the physical constituents, (2) perspiration in terms of excretions, (3) eyes in terms of the sensory organs, (4) liver in terms of the vital organs, and (5) gall bladder and small intestines in terms of the reservoir organs.

Phlegm disorders mainly course in (1) the nutritional essence, flesh, fat, marrow, and essence of the regenerative fluid in terms of the physical constituents, (2) nose and tongue in terms of sensory organs, (3) feces and urine in terms of excretions, (4) lungs, spleen, and kidneys in terms of the five vital organs, and (5) stomach and urinary bladder in terms of the reservoir organs.

Time of Arising
The sixth of the nine branches on the diseased body trunk is the time of arising. It refers to the time when a disorder, after it has coursed through these pathways, arises and gradually manifests. There are nine leaves on this branch; these are natural factors that favor the arising of certain humors. The first three leaves — old age, adult, and child — refer to age group. A predominance of wind is found in aged persons as well as in those who are physically weak; thus, the first leaf is called old age, implying a predominance of wind.

A predominance of bile is found in adults as is indicated by the fact that usually an adult is more active, aggressive, and arrogant. Thus, the second leaf is called the adult, implying a predominance of bile.

Phlegm is predominant in small children who by virtue of their age are physically weak. Thus, the third leaf is the child, implying a predominance of phlegm. During these three periods of life, there is greater danger from diseases associated with the predominant age-linked humor — wind problems in old age, bile problems in mid-life, and phlegm problems as a child.

Then, there are three leaves in terms of how locality — the nature of the place where one lives — favors the occurrence of a predominance of a certain humor. An area that is high in altitude and cold and thus where there is much cool wind, leads to an increase of wind in persons living there. In a place that is dry and hot, bile naturally increases. In a low, humid location, phlegm naturally increases.

The last three leaves on the time of arising branch are concerned with seasonal and temporal factors that favor the arising of particular humors. Wind disorders usually arise or increase — in terms of the day — at dawn and in the early evening; thus a sign that a person has a wind disorder is that symptoms are worse at dawn and in the early evening. In terms of season, wind disorders predominantly arise during the monsoon.

Symptoms of bile disorders are most manifest during the middle of the day and the middle of the night. The season that promotes bile disorders is autumn. Phlegm disorders mainly occur during spring, and their symptoms arise in stronger form early in the morning and at dusk.

Fatal Effects
The next branch is the resultant or effect branch, which has nine leaves. It is concerned with terminal situations that are such that from the very beginning the patient has to engage in religious techniques to accumulate merit and purify ill-

deeds, for once a bad karma that would cut short a life has been accumulated and once it ripens into fruition, it cannot be overcome by techniques such as material medicine.

Three causes are needed to sustain physical life — a life span established by former actions, merit, and good karma; these three have to work together. Life is not sustained just by good food and good behavior patterns; if such were the case, then prosperous persons living in a clean environment, as is often the case in the West, would necessarily live very long lives, but this is not so.

Life span, merit, and good karma; these are hard to understand because they involve religious topics. For instance, in order to have a long lifespan, it must be that, in the former lifetime during which you accumulated the karma impelling this life, you did not commit murder and protected the lives of others. Also, merit refers to having respected altruistic behavior, engaged in charity, and so forth. In this context karma refers to other types of virtuous actions and to refraining from non-virtuous actions.

Therefore, the first leaf on the fatal effects branch consists of the three main factors that terminate life: exhaustion of life span, karma, and merit. For, when these three factors are exhausted, the disorder is fatal. Though this topic is difficult at first to understand, if you look into it, it becomes clearer and clearer since it is founded in the actual situation of our lives.

The second leaf is the non-acceptance of the treatment applied. Even though the correct treatment for a particular disorder is given, the disorder does not respond, and the very medicine that usually cures it even aggravates the situation — the medicine increases the disease. In such cases, again, the disorder proves fatal; the problem is that one's karma has been exhausted.

Similarly, the third leaf on the effect branch is non-effectiveness of diet, medication, behavior patterns, and accessory therapy — a lack of response to these. The fourth leaf is fatal injury to a vital organ, essential for the maintenance of life. If an organ such as the brain, heart, or liver, is struck with a weapon such as an arrow, a sharp stone, knife, and so forth, the effect could be critical and not susceptible to cure.

The fifth leaf on the fatal effect branch is the termination of the life wind; this means that the power of the life-sustaining wind has become exhausted. The time of possible treatment has passed, and thus in spite of any efforts, the disorder proves fatal.

The sixth leaf is excessively advanced heat diseases. These are heat disorders that are terminal due to having passed beyond the point of effective treatment. The next leaf is excessively advanced cold disorders that are beyond treatment, not having been treated when they first arose and while still susceptible to medication, etc. Again, the disorder proves fatal.

The eighth leaf refers to cases when medication is ineffective because the physical constituents have become so depleted that they are not able to accept treatment. The body is so weak that it is at odds with the force of the medicine.

Finally, the ninth leaf is possession by a spirit such that the life force has been stolen away. As before, these are extreme, incurable cases since the topic is fatal effects, mortal situations.

Side Effects
The eighth branch, side effects, has twelve leaves. The first leaf is production of bile side effects during successful treatment of a wind disorder. The second leaf is production of phlegm side effects during successful treatment of wind disorders. These two are cases of the wind medicine's being too strong.

The third leaf is the production of bile side effects during unsuccessful treatment of wind disorders; the fourth is the production of phlegm side effects during unsuccessful treatment of wind disorders. In these two cases the wind medicine is of insufficient potency, resulting in imbalances in bile or phlegm. From these first four, you can understand the remaining eight.

The fifth is the production of wind side effects during successful treatment of bile disorders. The sixth is production of phlegm side effects during successful treatment of bile disorders. The seventh is production of wind side effects during ineffective treatment of bile disorders, and the eighth, production of phlegm side effects during ineffective treatment of bile disorders.

The ninth is production of wind side effects during successful treatment of phlegm disorders; the tenth, production of bile side effects during successful treatment of phlegm disorders. The eleventh is production of wind side effects during ineffective treatment of phlegm disorders, and the twelfth, production of bile side effects during ineffective treatment of phlegm disorders.

To avoid these side effects, medications must be of proper potency and contain supportive medications to avoid promoting imbalances in other humors.

Condensation
The ninth branch, a condensation of all diseases, has two leaves, cold and hot. This means that basically all disorders can be condensed into two categories: cold and hot. Wind and phlegm ailments are said to have a nature of coolness, like water; thus they are classified as cold disorders. Blood and bile ailments have a nature of heat, like fire; thus they are classified as hot disorders.

Apart from these, ailments involving organisms or lymph are common to both. If organisms or lymph are accompanied by a predominance of wind or phlegm, the disease is to be put in the cold category whereas if they are accompanied by a predominance of blood or bile, the disease is classed as a heat disorder.

4 Wind, Bile, And Phlegm

Let us return to the first trunk — the healthy body — which has three branches — the humors, the physical constituents, and the excretions. The three humors are wind, bile, and phlegm, each of which is divided into five major categories, yielding fifteen types of humors, these being the fifteen leaves on the humor branch.[14] I will explain the location of these fifteen humors, their area of function, and then their functions.

WIND

The life-sustaining wind is located at the crown of the head, and it mainly courses from that area through the chest. With respect to its functions, it enables the swallowing of food, inhalation, spitting out saliva, burping, and sneezing. It provides clarity to one's mind and to the sense organs and holds life in the sense that it provides the physical basis for the mind.

The location of the ascending wind is the breastbone. It courses or functions principally around the nose, tongue, and throat. Its functions are that it enables speech, provides physical strength and tone, empowers effort in the sense of stimulating activity, and gives clarity of memory and attention.

The pervasive or diffusive wind has its location in the heart. Though its basic site is the heart, it pervades every part of the body. Its functions are to perform flexion and extension of the limbs and the opening and closing of the apertures of the body such as the mouth, eyes, and so forth. Thus, most muscular actions are controlled by the pervasive wind.

The fire-accompanying wind has its locus in the lower part of the stomach and courses through all the hollow places — the intestines, gall bladder, channels in the heart, and so forth. Its functions are that it helps digestion, or metabolism, in the sense of ripening nourishment and separating refined and unrefined portions, and it consequently develops the respective colors of blood, bile, and so forth. The stomach is divided into three parts: the top is the location of the decomposing phlegm; the central part is where the digestive bile works, and the lower part is where the fire-accompanying wind works, so called because it is involved in the process of digestion which is like fire.

The downwards-voiding wind is located in the region of the genitals. It functions throughout the lower abdomen — the large intestine, urinary bladder, genitals, and thighs. Its functions are to control the mechanism of releasing and retaining semen, menses, feces, and urine. It also holds the fetus in the womb and releases the fetus in childbirth.

That is the way the medical system describes the locations, area of function, and functions of the five winds. Regarding the location of the life-sustaining wind and the pervasive wind, the tantric systems of the Old and New Translation Schools differ. The New Translation Schools reverse their locations, putting the life-sustaining wind at the heart and the pervasive wind at the crown of the head. The Old Translation School, however, is as was described above. Though the locations differ, their respective functions are the same.

Besides the five major types of wind there are five secondary winds. These can be divided into many more aspects and categories, but here we have just treated the five major ones.

Question: Are these winds the breath functioning throughout the body, or something more subtle?
Answer: Here wind does not refer to just breath but to factors that control breathing and many other things. Thus, it is different from breath itself, though it has a correspondence in terms of its characteristics. Wind is rough, light, cold, subtle, hard, and motile.

Since wind is one of the five elements, it is important to understand the lay-out of the five elements. This round world is constituted by the elements of earth, water, fire, wind, and space, and sentient beings' bodies also have the nature of these same five elements. Thus, blood and bile have a nature of fire; phlegm has a nature of earth and water; wind is that which moves these.

Now, without earth, there would be no basis or foundation. Without water, things would not cohere. Without fire, things could not mature or ripen. Without wind, things could not grow and increase. Without space, there would be no opportunity or place for things to grow. You should understand the humors within the context of the five elements. The external environment is composed of the five elements, and the beings inhabiting that environment are also composed of the same five elements; hence, the structure of the two is the same.

Humans experience six tastes — sweet, sour, bitter, astringent, hot, and salty — which are determined by the predominance of the five elements. A carrot, for instance, is produced in terms of the five elements. Earth (or hardness) provides the foundation; water acts as a cohesive factor, that is, it holds the carrot together. Fire is the factor enabling it to ripen and mature. The air or wind element enables it to grow, and the space element gives it the opportunity to manifest and to develop. In a carrot, earth and water are predominant, producing a sweet taste, and thus when a carrot is ingested, it will increase strength in the body.

Question: Of the characteristics of wind, are not rough and subtle contradictory?
Answer: Rough and subtle as qualities of wind are not contradictory. Rough is opposite to smooth, whereas subtle here denotes the capacity to move everywhere.

Question: Is wind the same as nerve impulses?
Answer: It's not quite the same. Wind controls nerve impulses.

Question: What wind controls the circulation of blood in the body?
Answer: The circulation of blood depends specifically upon the pervasive wind and the fire-accompanying wind. The fire-accompanying wind courses in all the hollow parts of the body, such as the nerves, blood vessels, and so forth.

Question: How is the predominance of a particular humor known in an individual?
Answer: Basically, there are two ways to perceive things validly: one by direct perception and another by inference. The presence of the three humors in the human body can be inferred. For instance, if a person's skin is rough, you can infer from this that the person has a high level of wind. Or, if a person experiences insomnia, you can infer that the person has a too high level of wind. Though the wind humor is not directly perceived, its presence can be inferred from symptoms, just as the presence of fire can be known from perceiving smoke, a sign of fire.

BILE
The bile humor, having a nature of fire, also consists of five

types. The first and most important is the digestive bile; it is very influential. Its location is in the stomach between the not yet digested and already digested food, that is, in the middle of the stomach. Its functions are that, like fire, it ripens or digests food, separates the refined and unrefined portions of food, produces bodily heat, activates and assists the other four biles, and provides bodily strength.

Next is the color-regulating bile. Its locus is mainly in the liver, but it functions throughout the body. It regulates color in the seven physical constituents — nutritional essence, blood, flesh, fat, bone, marrow, and regenerative fluid. For instance, it makes blood red, bone white, bile yellow, fingernails clear, and so forth.

Third is the determining or achieving bile. Its locus is at the heart, and its functions are to provide determination, decisiveness, and self-confidence in performing actions and in accomplishing your desires, preventing discouragement. In a negative way, it causes generation of overly assertive states of mind, such as pride.

The fourth type is the seeing bile, responsible for sight. Located in the eyes, it enables you to see.

The last, the complexion-clearing bile, is located in the skin; it provides skin tone, a good complexion.

The characteristics of bile — which basically has a nature of fire — are oiliness, sharpness, pungency (hotness), lightness, possessing a strong odor, a purgative quality, and moistness.

PHLEGM

Phlegm is also of five types. The first is the supportive phlegm, located along the breastbone. Its main function is to provide moisture throughout the body, such as saliva in the mouth, but it also provides cohesion, that is, holds the body together and provides support for the other four types of phlegm.

Next is the decomposing phlegm, located in the first part of the stomach, where the undigested food first localizes. Its main function is to mix and decompose the food that has been ingested.

The experiencing phlegm is located in the tongue. Its function is to provide the capacity for taste of the six types — sweet, sour, salty, bitter, hot, and astringent.

The satisfying phlegm, located in the brain, brings satisfaction. For instance, when the eyes see an object or the ears hear a sound, it is that factor which brings satisfaction. It also provides for deciding, for instance, that a taste is sweet or sour, that an odor is fragrant or not, that a sound is pleasant or unpleasant, that a form is good or bad, etc.

Finally, the connective phlegm, located in all the large and small joints, functions in connecting the joints and enabling flexion and extension.

Phlegm has the characteristics of oiliness, coolness, heaviness, bluntness, firmness, smoothness, and stickiness. Altogether there are twenty characteristics of the three humors.

Question: Do people tend to be dominated by one of the humors?
Answer: Persons can be classified on the basis of a natural humoral predominance into seven groups — those having a natural predominance of wind, bile, or phlegm singly; a double combination; and a triple combination. Thus, there are persons having a wind nature, a bile nature, a phlegm nature, a wind-bile nature, a wind-phlegm nature, a phlegm-bile nature, or a wind-bile-phlegm nature.

Question: Are these types of people distinguishable by physical observation?
Answer: A physician can distinguish those with a single predominance easily through physical observation even without seeing the urine or reading the pulse. The double combinations are more difficult, and the triple combination is very difficult to determine. The texts identify these types in detail.

Question: What is the difference between the oiliness of phlegm and of bile? Also, what is the difference between the oiliness and the stickiness of phlegm?

Answer: The difference between the oiliness of phlegm and of bile is that phlegm has a greasiness or oiliness on a superficial level whereas it ultimately does not have an oily nature. Bile, on the other hand, has oiliness in its very nature as well as an oily appearance. Stickiness is neither a dry or wet quality, but refers to a factor of adherability when touched.

Question: What is the relationship between the phlegm we cough up and the humor phlegm?

Answer: The phlegm that we cough up does not result necessarily from having an excess of the humor phlegm though it is the main type; even without such an imbalance, one could still cough up phlegm due to bile or wind problems. Also, the coughing up of phlegm can come from an excessive potency of phlegm or from a deficiency in the potency of phlegm. The phlegm that we cough up and the humor phlegm are related in that they have a similar nature of earth and water.

The phlegm humor serves as the foundation of the body, providing the wet and moistening factors. The phlegm that is coughed up is largely due to an excess of the potency of phlegm. It works to maintain and sustain good health when it is in balance with other humors but produces disease when imbalanced.

5 Seven Physical Constituents

The next branch on the healthy body trunk is that of the physical constituents. As mentioned earlier, it has seven leaves: nutritional essence, blood, flesh, fat, bone, marrow, and regenerative fluid.

With respect to how the physical constituents are formed, through ingesting the six tastes of the five external elements in the form of food, etc., the five internal elements develop. The process of digestion, roughly speaking, takes place as follows. First, the ingested food passes down the gullet to the first part of the stomach, where the decomposing phlegm, one of the five types of phlegm, is located. Here the food is mixed, that is, liquid and solids are mixed together. Then it proceeds to the second part of the stomach, where the digestive bile is located. This bile breaks down the food further, and finally in the third part of the stomach, where the fire-accompanying wind is located, there is a separation of nutrients from waste products. The gross separation of wastes and nutrients begins at the third level of the stomach.

The seven physical constituents are produced at succeeding levels in this process as waste factors and nutrients (or unrefined and refined parts) are separated. The nutrients or constructive items are initially channeled to the liver, where blood is produced from them. Then, the nutritional essence of the blood is separated from the main blood and is transformed into flesh. Next, the nutritional essence (or refined part) of the flesh is transformed into fatty tissue, and then the nutritional essence of the fatty tissue is transformed into bone. The nutritional essence of the bones is transformed into marrow. Then the nutritional essence of the marrow is transformed into regenerative fluid.

With respect to the wastes (or unrefined parts), in the intestines the waste products that were separated from the nutrients in the third part of the stomach are transformed into solid and liquid forms. The solid turns into feces, and the liquid into urine, the latter being channeled to the urinary bladder.

The nutritional essence, extracted in the third part of the stomach, is, as was said before, transformed into blood by the liver. The waste products of that nutritional essence act as factors assisting the decomposing phlegm in the first part of the stomach. The waste products of the blood are channeled to the gall bladder. The waste matter of the flesh produces the excretions from the nine openings in the body, such as wax in the ears and the scum in the corners of the eyes. The waste matter of fatty tissue becomes body oil and perspiration. The waste products of the bone produce toenails, fingernails, and hair. The waste part of the marrow produces the basic oiliness of the skin and flesh. The oiliness mentioned earlier in connection with fat is a greasiness that, if washed, can be removed; here, the oiliness produced from the waste products of the marrow is inherent or natural oiliness that cannot be removed by washing.

The non-nutrient or waste part of the regenerative fluid turns into semen — the fluid that can produce a child. The final, purest part of the regenerative fluid is localized at the heart, though it is present in all parts of the body. This nutrient or refined part of the regenerative fluid sustains life, determines one's life span, and provides a bright complexion and physical tone.

Generally, the period required for the entire digestive cycle from the ingestion of food to the production of the regenerative fluid to take place is six or seven days. However, there are certain types of medications that do not follow this sequence; some fertility drugs are transformed in a short time, even less than a day, from the state of nutritional essence into regenerative fluid without passing through the other parts of the cycle. Also, some foods bypass parts of the sequence. In these cases the cycle of digestion takes less than the normal period of six to seven days.

This has been a rough explanation of how the process of digestion takes place. Each of these transformations can be explained in much greater detail.

CONCLUSION OF THE HEALTHY BODY TRUNK

The third and final branch on the healthy body trunk is the excretions — factors that cannot be assimilated and need to be expelled from the body. It has only three leaves: feces, urine, and perspiration. These require no further explanation.

Thus, altogether there are twenty-five leaves growing on the three branches of the first trunk (healthy body) on the first root (body). They are present even in a healthy body, and it is on this basis that they have been explained.

A healthy body is defined as a state of balance of the twenty-five leaves or categories and food and behavior patterns. Life-increasing health free from disease exists when there is harmony or balance among the twenty-five factors, the tastes and power of the food ingested, and behavior patterns. That concludes the outline of the first trunk, the healthy body.

6 Causes, Conditions, and Entrances

The second trunk is the diseased body. As was mentioned before, the first branch on the unhealthy body trunk is that of cause — the distant cause being beginningless ignorance. The more proximate causes — wind, bile, and phlegm — derive from, or have their psychological base in, three negative states of mind — desire, hatred, and obscuration. The latter, which themselves originate from the basis of all disorders, ignorance, are the three leaves on the cause branch.

In dependence upon desire, hatred, and obscuration, there arise, respectively, increases of wind, bile, and phlegm. The disorders associated with the three humors can be classified, as mentioned before, into forty-two types of wind disorders, twenty-six types of bile disorders, and thirty-three types of phlegm disorders.

These 101 humoral disorders are derived from a broader classification of 1,616 disorders which itself can be seen as a condensation of 84,000 types of disorders, corresponding with 84,000 types of afflictive states of mind. In other words, in correspondence with 84,000 negative states of mind, there are 84,000 disorders which can be classified or condensed into 1,616, which can be further classified as

404, which again are condensed into 101 types of disorders on the basis of humoral imbalance.

Diseases are classified in another way into three types according to their causes. The first are those caused by mere disturbance or imbalance among the humors in this lifetime. The second are caused by actions committed in a past life, ripening in this life in the form of disorder. The third are caused by the presence of both factors, that is, imbalance of the three humors involving also maturation of a seed planted in a past lifetime by an action performed then.

Thus, the first of these three is called a one lifetime disorder, because an imbalance among the humors is created only by failure to observe proper diet and behavior patterns, and the cycle of the disease occurs in just one lifetime. The second type is known as a disorder resulting from a past life. Such diseases usually prove fatal, not responding to treatment because they involve the maturation of a negative action committed in a past life. Broadly speaking, the commission of the ten non-virtuous types of actions in a previous lifetime results in maturation in a future lifetime in the form of a disorder. The basic disease is rooted in the past.

Serious disorders, the evident cause of which is minor, are included in the third category — disorders caused by both factors, humoral imbalance in this life and the maturing of a seed implanted by an action committed in a past lifetime. Consequently, even though the evident cause may be of a minor nature, the disorder experienced can be severe.[15]

HUMORAL DISTURBANCE

When the three humors are in balance, health is maintained, disease being in a dormant state, but when an imbalance among the humors occurs, they become entities of disease, harming body and life and giving rise to suffering.[16] This means that once there is an imbalance, the foundations for harming the physical body, life span, and so forth are laid.

When a disorder of bile occurs, the seven physical constituents are heated. Bile is located in the lower part of the body, but when disturbed, it rises or spreads to the upper part of the body because of its nature of heat, or fire [which naturally rises upward]. All heat disorders have their origin in bile disturbances.

When a phlegm disorder occurs, it reduces or smothers bodily heat. Phlegm has a nature of earth and water and thus the qualities of heaviness and coolness; hence, though phlegm is located in the upper part of the body, it falls or descends to the lower part of the body. It is responsible for all cold disorders, that is, all cold disorders have their basis in the disturbance of phlegm.

Wind is common to both cold and heat; it assists whichever of the two, bile or phlegm, is more prominent. Thus, if a phlegm disturbance is prominent, wind acts to produce cold disorders. If a bile disturbance is prominent, wind aids the bile-disturbing factors and produces heat disorders. Wind pervades the entire body and promotes both heat and cold disorders.

CONDITIONS FOR DISEASE

The second branch of the diseased body trunk is the condition branch. With regard to the explanation of conditions,[17] a condition is defined as that factor enabling a cause to ripen and mature. There are three main types of conditions: (1) formation-increasing conditions which form an illness and increase it, (2) accumulation-arising conditions which collect an illness together and cause it to arise, and (3) manifesting conditions which cause the collected or stored illness to manifest.

Formation-Increasing Conditions
Formation-increasing conditions are of three types: (1) sea-

sons, (2) the sensory organs, and (3) behavior patterns. These three factors themselves are taught in terms of their being either deficient, excessive, or wrongly utilized. Three main seasons are mentioned in this context — the hot, cold, and rainy seasons. If the hot season is hotter or colder than what it normally should be, that excess or deficiency could act as a factor producing a disorder. The same is applied to cold and rainy seasons. Wrong utilization means to engage in a behavior pattern that does not correspond to the nature of the season; for instance, if during summer you wear excessively warm clothing, that is wrong utilization of the season.

Regarding sensory organs, if they are used excessively, too little, or wrongly, these very actions serve as factors to manifest disorders in the body. When the sensory organs come into contact with their respective objects, it is important to utilize this contact correctly because, for instance, if you gaze at a pleasant object or listen to pleasant sounds or smell fragrant odors more than is fitting, this could produce a disorder. Or, if you look at a frightful or repulsive object for too long a period or listen to unpleasant sounds too much, or smell bad odors too much, again this could be wrong utilization of the sensory organs and affect the humoral balance in the body. The same is true with tastes and objects of touch.

The idea is similar with regard to behavior patterns of body, speech, and mind. For instance, if you think or talk excessively, this could affect your state of health. Or if you overexercise, that could act as a factor to produce a disorder. Also, if you excessively withhold yourself from defecating or urinating or if when defecating or urinating you strain too much, this could serve as a formation-increasing condition for an illness.

Accumulation-Arising Conditions

Accumulation-arising conditions are discussed in three topics: accumulation, arising, and pacification in terms of causes, nature, and season. First, accumulation of the humors occurs, after which arising or manifestation occurs; these effects, however, can be pacified by other factors.

Causes. With respect to the causes of accumulation of a wind disease, for instance, wind is caused to accumulate in the body by the intake of food having characteristics corresponding to wind, basically foods that are rough and light such as tea or light and cool such as pork. Then, cold serves to cause the wind disease to arise. However, if you ingest food which has a warm or oily quality, then those characteristics prevent the accumulated wind from manifesting in the form of a disorder, thereby pacifying it.

If you take food items with hot and sharp qualities, such as hot pepper or liquor which is sharp and rough, or oily qualities, accumulation of bile occurs. Then, heat causes the bile disease to arise. However, if you take food with cool properties, the accumulation is prevented from arising, thus pacifying the manifestation of the disease. If you ingest food that causes bile to accumulate more than is required and opposing food properties do not subdue its arising, then an arising or manifestation takes place. Abnormal changes, therefore, can be prevented by taking balanced food.

Similarly with phlegm, if you take foods having the basic qualities or characteristics of phlegm, that is, heavy, oily, and cool properties, then phlegm accumulates in the body. Examples of foods with an oily nature are the different types of oils and animal fats. Potatoes have a heavy quality. Cauliflower, cabbage, and carrots have a cool quality. Then, warmth causes the phlegm disease to arise, like the heat of the sun melting ice. However, if you take rough and light food items, their qualities will help keep the disorder from arising.

The characteristics of a food item can be identified by tasting it. Taste serves as the best indicator of its composition in terms of the five elements, and from those elements, one can determine its properties — heaviness, coolness, and so forth. For instance, that the dominant elements of a carrot are water and earth can be inferred from its sweetness. From those elements its properties, its potencies, etc. can be determined. Earth has characteristics similar to phlegm — heaviness, compactness, stability, and stickiness. Water is moist, cool, blunt, smooth, and oily.

Nature. Accumulation is a normal process of the collection of wind, bile, and phlegm at the sites or locations of the respective humors. When manifestation of a disorder takes place, an abnormal process has been activated by conditions. When manifestation of what has been accumulated takes place, it can be inferred that an accumulated humor has left its original site and has diffused into other areas. Thus, manifestation or arising is an abnormal process, whereas accumulation is a normal process of digestion.

Season. In the astrological texts, there are five seasons: the four main seasons — spring, summer, autumn, and winter — each consisting of seventy-two days, and between each season there are inbetween seasons of eighteen days, altogether four sets of eighteen days. This yields a year of 360 days; [every fourth year has a leap month].

With respect to seasonal factors, earth and water predominate during winter; water and wood during spring; fire and wind during summer; iron and earth during fall; and earth during the inbetween seasons. The beginning of each of the four "Western" seasons corresponds to the middle of the four Tibetan seasons. Hence, the summer solstice when the sun is the farthest north is midsummer [rather than the beginning of the summer as in the "West"], and the winter solstice when the sun is the farthest south is midwinter [rather than the beginning of the winter as in the "West"]. In early summer the wind level increases; in late summer [the rainy season] bile increases, and in late winter phlegm increases. Thus, the accumulation or formation period for these three humors occurs at these times.

Wind. The reason why wind accumulates in early summer is that early summer is characterized by lightness and roughness. Since these seasonal characteristics correspond to the characteristics of wind, accumulation of wind takes place during this period. However, although accumulation takes place during early summer, this is not the time of the manifestation of wind disorders, because the heat of that season opposes the coolness of wind and thus prevents its arising; the wind disorder remains dormant.

During late summer the accumulated wind can manifest because late summer is the rainy season [in India] and thus cool and windy. The coolness activates the accumulated wind [which itself is cool] and causes it to manifest. Accumulation takes place at the original site of the humor; its manifestation means that it has exceeded what the normal site can hold, and it now seeks other pathways.

Even if abnormal dislocation of wind has occurred, a natural pacification of wind can take place in autumn because autumn has the characteristics of being warm [after the end of the rainy season] and of being oily. These characteristics help to subdue or control manifested wind. "Oily" refers to a predominant quality in autumn that helps to subdue the light and mobile nature of wind which has manifested.

Bile. During late summer [the rainy season] the accumulation of bile takes place because of the oily nature of that period. However, because of its cool characteristic which opposes the heat of bile, manifestation cannot take place.

In autumn the manifestation or arising of bile occurs because of the characteristic oiliness and warmth of fall [since the rains have ended]. During winter, pacification of the manifestation of bile disorders occurs due to the cool nature of the season.

Phlegm. During the late part of winter accumulation of phlegm occurs because of the heavy, cold, and oily characteristics of that part of the year. Because of the very cold characteristic of the season, the phlegm is, so to speak, frozen; then during early spring the heat of the sun melts the "frozen" phlegm, allowing the arising of phlegm disorders through its diffusion into regions or pathways other than its original site. However, because of the very hot, light, and rough characteristics of early summer, pacification of phlegm disorders can naturally take place.

This explains how the pacification of manifestation occurs naturally in the body due to seasonal factors, without resorting to external methods.

Manifesting Conditions

Nevertheless, if a person takes improper diet and engages in improper behavior patterns, the process of accumulation and arising in terms of the seasons need not be involved. A disorder of any of the humors can manifest in any season due to improper diet, improper behavior, and a person's natural disposition.

With respect to manifesting conditions, there are two: general and specific. General manifesting conditions, which cause imbalance of the humors, are improper diet, improper behavior patterns, spirits, seasonal factors [as just described], improper medication, poison, and fruition of negative actions.

Specific manifesting conditions are the specific ways that the general conditions function to cause manifestation of disorders of the three humors individually. Conditions for the arising of wind disorders include overconsumption of anything — food, drink, or medicine — that has a bitter taste or is light and rough in nature. These will cause wind disorders to manifest, as will much desire (particularly sexual desire but also other desires), going hungry, sleeplessness, excessive verbal and physical activities particularly on an empty stomach (thus if in the morning on an empty stomach you engage in very strenuous activity such as exercise, this could cause wind disorders to arise), bleeding (the loss of blood gives an opportunity for wind to diffuse into these regions), vomiting or diarrhea (which weaken the body, giving a good opportunity for the light quality of the wind humor to form), exposure to cool breezes, generation of excessive joy, sadness, or much weeping when an event takes place, mental depression (for instance, from failing to accomplish something or from obsession), intake of much non-nutritious food, exertion in defecating, and exertion in retaining urine or stool.

To repeat, the factors or the conditions that cause accumulated wind disorders suddenly to manifest are as follows. If you take an excessive quantity of food with a bitter taste or having a light and rough power, this will aggravate accumulated wind. For instance, taking too much coffee or strong tea or foods such as cucumber aggravate wind as they have a light and rough power. Also pork aggravates accumulated wind because it is cool and light. However, if you take these in a moderate quantity, they will not be harmful; only when you take them in excessive quantity are they injurious.

In terms of behavior patterns, generation of excessive desire — particularly for sex but also for material objects, going hungry for a long period of time, lack of sleep, engaging in strenuous activities such as exercise on an empty stomach, excessive talking, much bleeding, much vomiting, and strong diarrhea provide conditions for accumulated wind to manifest. With regard to desire, when you are attached to an object, think a lot about trying to get it, and then do not attain it, the resultant tension can upset accumulated wind.

Exposure to breezes for too long a period causes wind aggravation, as does generation of excessive pleasure or joy in reaction to an event or severe depression and crying for a long period of time. Also, excessively using the mind provides an opportunity for accumulated wind to manifest. Eating non-nutritious food frequently does the same. For instance, potatoes, peas, and beans are non-nutritious food items, particularly if taken after discarding the water in which they are cooked. They should be cooked in just enough water so that the water is used up in the cooking process; baked potatoes are more nutritious. Also, potatoes are cool in nature and not very nutritious; thus, taken just on their own without butter or other foods, they are classified as non-nutritious.

Again, either forceful retention or forceful expelling of feces, urine, or mucus from the body, as well as excessively forceful sneezing or spitting are harmful. They create an environment where wind can easily be aggravated.

Regarding the specific manifesting conditions that cause the manifestation of bile after it has accumulated, if you take too much food that is hot, sharp, salty, or oily, bile disorders can manifest. In terms of mental attitude, if you generate hatred and associated negative states of mind, bile rises above its normal accumulation. Also, sleeping during a very hot afternoon and then working hard aggravates accumulated bile so that it spreads to parts of the body other than its normal sites. Also, strenuous activities, such as carrying a very heavy object beyond one's capacity, pulling the string of a tight bow, wrestling, running, becoming excessively tired due to moving about and working during the heat of the day, being thrown off a horse, falling off a cliff, or being beaten can aggravate accumulated bile.

Food items such as very nutritious meat, butter, molasses, beer, and so forth — anything producing excessive heat — can cause accumulated bile to manifest as a disease if taken in excessive quantity.

To repeat, the principal factors creating the conditions for accumulated bile to manifest are as follows. Excessive intake of foods which have the following qualities: in terms of taste, a hot taste and in terms of power, a sharp and oily power. Sharp and hot food items are, for instance, any type of pepper. An oily food item would be any oil, particularly those extracted from grains.

Regarding behavior patterns, if you generate excessive hatred toward something or someone, this mental factor causes manifestation of bile already accumulated in the body. Sleeping during the daytime, particularly after lunch on a hot day, causes aggravation of bile, as does engaging in strenuous physical activity — for instance, trying to carry a particularly heavy object. Shoveling and digging in hard ground are also harmful this way as is pulling hard on the string of a bow. These types of physical strain place tremendous tension in the body, thereby causing the aggravation of bile. The same is true of hard running or jogging for a long time with a sense of intense competitiveness. Being thrown off a horse, falling off a cliff, playing rough sports, being buried underground such as under sand, or being beaten by a stick do the same.

If you take too much mutton or yak meat, that is harmful to bile because these meats are very hot and also have a heavy quality. Likewise are butter, molasses, and liquor such as whiskey — beer is not so harmful because it has a cooler quality than liquor. The more time it takes to process an alcoholic drink, the more harmful it is in terms of aggravating bile and the more curative power it has in terms of phlegm. Hence, in phlegm disorders, the older the wine or liquor is, the better, whereas in the case of bile it is the other way around. The main point is that if you take more of these foods and drinks than the body can naturally absorb, they become harmful, causing manifestation of bile disorders.

Now we come to the factors that cause manifestation of phlegm disorders. In terms of food items, these are mainly any that are sweet in taste or heavy, cool, or oily in nature. If foods having these characteristics are taken in excess of what is required for normal balance, phlegm diffusion occurs. Flour and mutton are heavy. Pork has a very cool quality, as do oranges and sugar. Wheat flour is heavy and cool and thus helpful to wind and bile but harmful to phlegm. Cauliflower and cabbage are heavy and sweet and thus harmful for accumulated phlegm; in terms of taste they are sweet, and in terms of potency, heavy. Staying immobile particularly after a heavy meal — some movement but not heavy exercise being preferable — or sleeping during the day can also aggravate accumulated phlegm.

The natural predominance of the humors must be considered. For instance, if the person concerned has a strong predominance of wind by nature, a short nap after meals is recommended to balance the natural wind predominance. However, if the person has a natural predominance of phlegm, sleeping after a meal would only aggravate it further.

Sleeping in a moist place aggravates phlegm, as does exposure to cold after a cold shower or bath. Also uncooked grains, such as wheat or corn, and uncooked peas and so forth as well as unripe fruit aggravate phlegm. The taste of unripened fruit is sour, and because it is not fully ripened, its full power has not manifested, whereby it has a heavy quality. Those two factors — sourness and heaviness — mean that when ingested, it aggravates phlegm because of the correspondence of qualities between the unripened fruit and phlegm.

Goat meat and the flesh or fat of thin cattle also contribute to the manifestation of phlegm disorders. The oils of grains such as mustard, peanut, corn, and sunflower oil as well as rancid butter promote the manifestation of phlegm disorders. Also, raw vegetables such as carrots, cabbage, or lettuce aggravate phlegm, as does wild mountain garlic and so forth. Also, any food that is overcooked, uncooked, undercooked, burned, or cooked but taken cold is harmful to phlegm. Although cow's milk and yogurt are cool and light in nature, goat's milk and yogurt are cool, heavy, and sweet and thus harmful to phlegm. Their post-digestive taste is also sweet, due to which these promote organisms particularly in the abdomen.

Cold tea and cold water also aggravate phlegm, as do overeating or overdrinking. Finally, if you eat food before the previous meal has been digested — especially in the case of having eaten heavy, oily foods — and if you do this over a considerable period of time, this will decrease the fires of digestion and act as a factor to increase phlegm and aggravate accumulated phlegm. In short, these factors cause the aggravation or manifestation of phlegm after it has accumulated in its normal way.

It should be remembered that the body has a tremendous capacity to adapt to the ingestion of various foods. Particularly, the foods eaten as a child are often very digestible and beneficial since you are so used to them.

Question: What about preservatives and additives?
Answer: Each substance on earth naturally has its own potency. Thus, additives and preservatives have their own qualities, and if, for example, an additive with a coarse potency is added to food that is by nature coarse, it could be harmful. These substances increase or decrease the natural powers of the food item. In Tibet after the introduction of fertilizers, although grain grown with the help of fertilizers grew in much larger quantity, it was less nutritious; grain grown without fertilizers was more beneficial.

Question: Are there certain foods that should not be mixed, certain foods that when mixed will cause problems?
Answer: For instance, if you eat fungus grown on trees that has been fried in mustard oil, that would be very toxic. Food poisoning could also result from cooking chicken and fish together in the same container; it does not cause immediate death as some poisons do but brings about harm

internally. Chicken is light whereas fish is heavy.

In another case, if you cook any type of peas or beans with molasses or brown sugar, that immediately produces a toxic quality. Worse still, if yogurt is taken with this, it becomes very poisonous by increasing certain organisms in the body inordinately.

Question: Do you know about these toxic effects only theoretically through combinations of qualities of foods as determined by taste or do you know them through observation of toxic reactions in patients without any reference to theory?

Answer: These are known both from the nature of the foods and from their having occurred in the past. Buddha's knowledge is non-delusive [and thus his explanation of the nature of foods is without error]. For instance, chicken is light and fish is heavy; thus, if these two are cooked in the same vessel, they conflict with each other. The determination is made by way of careful consideration of their tastes and potencies; there is no harm if chicken and fish are eaten together; the harm comes in cooking them in the same vessel.

With this we conclude the branch of conditions. On the unhealthy body trunk we have covered the first two of the nine branches — causes and conditions.

ENTRANCE BRANCH

The third branch on the unhealthy body trunk is the entrances of illnesses.[18] It has six leaves — skin, flesh, channels, bone, vital organs, and reservoir organs — telling how after the causes of disorders are activated by conditions, the process of a disease passes through various parts of the body, diffusing and localizing.

This topic is generally taught in terms of the six entrances, but the order is not absolute. Diseases of the three humors spread in the *skin*, develop in the *flesh*, move in the *vessels*, form in the *bones*, descend into the *vital organs*, and finally fall into the *reservoir organs*.[19]

The main site of wind is the bones. The main sites of bile are blood and perspiration. Phlegm is mainly in the remaining physical constituents.

The three humors are interdependent. Phlegm, being of a nature of earth and water, acts as the foundation of the humors because it has a heavy quality; bile, having a nature of fire, functions on the foundation laid by phlegm; and wind, having a nature of motility, works with both phlegm and bile to keep them going. Without any one of them, health and life are not possible. They are interdependent, and consequently any disturbance of these three affects the seven physical constituents and then the three excretions. This is the general sequence of how a disturbance affects one factor and then the next.

With respect to how disorders first enter the body solely in terms of improper diet, when you ingest a food that has similar characteristics to one of the humors, the pervasive wind diffuses the food particles to all cavities of the body. Possibly because of a humoral disfunction, one of these pathways could be blocked, meaning that the food in its first form — the first of the physical constituents, nutritional essence — would be confined to a particular area more than is required. Because of this blockage, excess localization takes place, and just as a dark cloud ultimately means a heavy shower over the spot where it appears, this blockage and formation of the nutritional essence at this specific place due to blockage means that severe accumulation and finally manifestation of a corresponding humoral disorder will occur when the appropriate conditions for arising are met. It is from this point that the topic of the entrances applies.

With respect to the more specific pathways of humoral disorders,[20] the wind humor spreads in the hips and all the joints of the body in terms of the parts of the body, in the skin and the ears in terms of the senses, and particularly in the lower part of the stomach and the large intestine in terms of the vital and the reservoir organs. These are the specific places or locations where accumulated wind primarily manifests.

Bile diseases usually are located in the stomach, the blood, perspiration, nutritional essence, lymph, the eyes, the skin, and principally the middle part of the stomach.

Phlegm diseases are mainly located in the chest, throat region, lungs, head, nutritional essence, flesh, fatty tissue, marrow, regenerative fluid, feces, urine, nose, tongue, and principally the first part of the stomach.

The remaining branches on the diseased body trunk will not be explained further because the earlier descriptions of these branches and leaves suffice for our purposes here. Now, we will pass on to the diagnostic root — the methods of diagnosis.

PART TWO

DIAGNOSIS

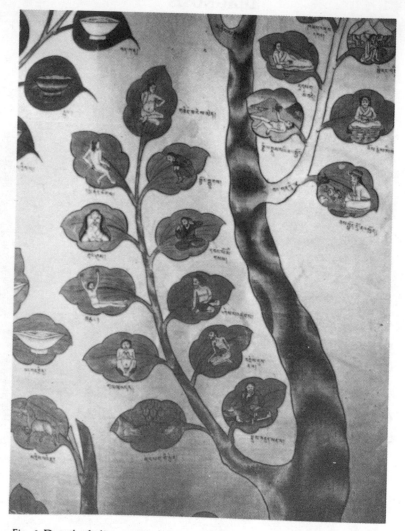

Fig. 3 Detail of the medicine tree which focuses on leaves from the questioning trunk.

DIAGNOSIS ROOT

3 Trunks, 8 Branches, 38 Leaves

VISUAL OBSERVATION TRUNK

(1) *Tongue Observation Branch*
  1. Wind Tongue
  2. Bile Tongue
  3. Phlegm Tongue

(2) *Urine Observation Branch*
  1. Wind Urine
  2. Bile Urine
  3. Phlegm Urine

PULSE FEELING TRUNK

(1) *Wind Pulse Branch*
  1. Wind Pulse Beat

(2) *Bile Pulse Branch*
  1. Bile Pulse Beat

(3) *Phlegm Pulse Branch*
  1. Phlegm Pulse Beat

QUESTIONING TRUNK

(1) *Wind Questioning Branch*
  Causal Conditions:
  1. Coarse food, tea, pork, goat's meat, staying in cool breezes
  Symptoms:
  2. Yawning and Shivering
  3. Sighing and stretching limbs frequently
  4. Cold chills
  5. Aches in hips, waist, bones, joints
  6. Uncertain moving pain
  7. Dry heaves

  8. Dulling of sense organs
  9. Mental roughness, restlessness
  10. Hunger pains
  Remedies:
  11. Greasy, nutritious food, warm place, close friends

(2) *Bile Questioning Branch*
  Causal Conditions:
  1. Sharp, hot food, vigorous conduct, sitting in sun
  Symptoms:
  2. Bitter taste in mouth
  3. Frequent headaches
  4. Surface fever
  5. Aches in upper body
  6. Digestive pain
  Remedies:
  7. Cool food (e.g., yogurt) and cool conduct (such as sitting by seashore)

(3) *Phlegm Questioning Branch*
  Causal Conditions:
  1. Heavy, greasy food, sitting or lying on ground
  Symptoms:
  2. Loss of appetite
  3. Fullness of stomach even without eating
  4. Frequent vomiting
  5. Heaviness of mind and body
  6. Indigestion
  7. Frequent belching
  8. No sense of taste
  9. Coldness in mind and body
  10. Discomfort after eating
  Remedies:
  11. Hot food and conduct (sitting by fire, sitting in sun, wearing warm clothing)

7 Pulse 1

First I will describe the method of diagnosis by touch, feeling the pulse, because it is supreme among methods of diagnosis.[21] It has three branches: wind, bile, and phlegm pulses. The textbook in which pulse diagnosis is explained is the fourth, the *Last Tantra*, in the first of twenty-five chapters.

As explained earlier, the teaching was requested by a manifestation of the Medicine Buddha's speech and was set forth by Amoghasiddhi. The first chapter of the *Last Tantra* has thirteen sections, explaining the various aspects and nature of pulse diagnosis. The first section deals with the requirements of diet and behavior that persons whose pulse is to be taken have to observe the day before the pulse is read as well as requirements for the physician to observe before reading the pulse of a patient. The second section explains the time when pulse diagnosis should be done. The third deals with the place for pulse diagnosis — the parts of the body where pulse can be read most effectively. The fourth is concerned with the amount of pressure to be applied at the place where the pulse is read. The remaining sections describe how to take the pulse, the three classes of constitutional pulses, seasonal effects on pulse, divination pulses, differences in pulse beats in health and disease, general and specific pulses, death pulses, spirit pulses, and life span pulse.

PREREQUISITE DIET AND BEHAVIOR

First, let us describe the behavior and dietary patterns to be observed by physician and patient before the process of pulse reading.[22] These have particular importance in terms of the description later, in the eighth section, of the seven wondrous or amazing pulses which are used to foretell various events. The Tibetan system of pulse taking is divided into two types — diagnostic and prognostic — and the first section on prerequisites is particularly important in determining prognostic pulses.

Except in emergencies, it is recommended that the doctor defer the pulse reading and advise the patient to follow a certain diet for at least one day before the pulse is read. Patients are advised not to take any food that is extremely nutritious or very warming, such as a large quantity of meat, butter, or alcohol, and to avoid any food difficult to digest including cold foods — in short, any type of food that would affect the humors in the body in an unusual way. Also, patients should neither go hungry nor overeat, nor eat food to which they are not habituated, in that it may be difficult to digest. They should not engage in any sexual activity during the day prior to reading the pulse. Also, they should not perform any strenuous activity, particularly on an empty stomach, nor go without sleep, nor talk too much, worry, or argue.

These dietary and behavior patterns also apply to the physician.

TIME OF PULSE READING

The best time to read the pulse is early in the morning, at dawn when one first can see the lines on the palm of the hand.[23] The text describes this as when the sun first appears, but its rays do not strike the plains, just the hills. One should read the pulse at that time because the day and night energy rhythms of the body are in balance. The hot, sun rhythm and the cold, moon rhythm are most balanced at this time. During this pre-sunrise period, the warm breath has not been exhaled in large quantity, and the cold air has not been greatly inhaled. Because the wind patterns are in balance, except for emergencies a doctor would choose to read the pulse of a patient at this time. The patient should not have taken food.

PLACE OF PULSE READING

The best place for reading the pulse is about half an inch from the crease at the wrist, on the radial artery.[24] The index, middle, and ring fingers are to be placed in a straight line on the radial artery, half an inch from the crease of the wrist.[25] They should not touch each other but should also not be far apart — the distance between them being that of the width of a grain. Leaving a small space between them, place them in a straight line gently on the radial artery of the patient.

Question: Do you use any other pulse, such as the pulse of the throat?
Answer: Pulse can be read on any major artery of the body, for instance, at the neck, the heart, or elsewhere. However, it is primarily read on the radial artery, except in the case of determining what is called the death pulse; in that case it is read at the ankle. Except for that, in all cases the radial artery is chosen for reading the pulse because it is the most suitable artery in terms of accurately indicating the state of each of the organs since it is neither too near nor too far from them, a middle distance. From there you can pick up signs as to how each organ in the body is functioning.

Question: Is the death pulse taken when a disease is severe and the doctor wants to know if the patient is soon to die?

Or could it be taken on a healthy person to determine when that person will die?

Answer: The death pulse is taken in patients who are suffering from a severe and critical disorder such that it is just a matter of days until they will die. Physicians simply use it to determine the time the patient has left. Otherwise, in the case of a healthy patient, they use the seven wondrous pulses to determine the general life span of a person.

AMOUNT OF PRESSURE

Each of these three fingers are to exert varying pressure.[26] The first presses only the skin; the second one, enough to feel the flesh; and the third one, enough to feel the bone underneath it.

In the case of a female, the doctor examines her right arm first with his left hand. In the case of a male, first he examines the left arm with his right hand. Then, in each case he switches hands and examines the other arm of the patient.

The seats on which the doctor and patient sit should be of the same height. It is also important that the patient's breathing be normal; as we mentioned earlier, at dawn the hot breath and the cold breath are equal. Thus, that time is preferred.

HOW TO READ THE PULSE

First, as explained before, the fingers of the physician — smooth, sensitive, without scars, and pliant — should be placed on the radial artery in a straight line.[27] The heat of the doctor's fingertips should correspond to the bodily heat of the patient.

Again, in the case of a male patient, the left hand pulse is read first by the right hand of the physician. In the case of a female, the right hand pulse is read first by the left hand of the physician. The tips of the first three fingers of the physician's two hands are divided into two sections each, making altogether twelve divisions. Each of the divisions reads a specific major organ in the body. In terms of a male patient, on the index finger of the physician's right hand the upper division (the part nearer the thumb) reads the heart, and the lower division reads the small intestine. The upper division of the middle finger on the doctor's right hand reads the spleen; the lower division reads the stomach. The upper division of the ring finger reads the left kidney, and the lower division, the seminal vesicle.

The upper division of the index finger of the doctor's left hand reads the lungs, and the lower division of the index finger reads the large intestine. The upper division of the middle finger reads the liver; the lower, the gall bladder. The upper division of the ring finger reads the right kidney, and the lower division, the urinary bladder.

For female patients, the only difference is that the organs read by the index fingers are reversed. Thus, for a female patient the upper part of the doctor's right index finger reads the lungs, and the lower part, the large intestine. Also, the upper part of the left index finger reads the heart, and the lower, the small intestine. The reason for this switch is that the male has a predominance of the white constituent and thus the left channel, whereas the female has a predominance of the red constituent and thus the right channel. Consequently, the place where the mind initially enters the combination of blood and semen in the womb at the very beginning of this lifetime, this being where the heart initially forms, is slightly different for male and female.

CONSTITUTIONAL PULSES

Constitutional pulses refer to the fact that all persons possess certain categories of pulses, representing temperament and constitution.[28] They are read only when persons are in a healthy state for the sake of realizing the tendencies of an individual's natural physical constitution. There are three types of constitutional pulses having characteristics similar to the three humors; they are called male, female, and neuter or bodhisattva pulses. The male pulse is similar to wind; the female, to bile; and the bodhisattva or neuter, to phlegm. [The term "bodhisattva" here has no spiritual connotation.]

First, the male pulse beat is bulky and coarse. The female pulse is subtle and rapid. The bodhisattva pulse beat is long in continuum and smooth. "Long in continuum" means that the beat is gentle — a continual, slow beat. These three pulse beats do not have anything to do with one's gender.

If a male has a female pulse beat, that is, a subtle and rapid pulse beat, he will have a long life. If a female has a male pulse beat, bulky and coarse, she will give birth to children who have accumulated a lot of merit in past lives.

If both husband and wife have a bodhisattva, or neuter, pulse beat — a continual, slow, smooth pulse beat — both of them will have a long life, and disease will be rare during their life. Also, higher persons will be kind to them whereas those lower than they will be harsh; their uncles and aunts will act like enemies. They will be childless, and thus their family lineage will stop.

If both husband and wife have male pulse beats, they will have more sons than daughters. If both have female pulse beats, the number of daughters will be greater.

If one in the couple has a bodhisattva pulse and the other has a male pulse, they will have only one child, a male. If, on the other hand, one has a bodhisattva pulse beat and the other a female pulse, they will have only one child, a daughter.

It is important that the physician know a patient's constitutional pulse because, for instance, a male or female pulse beat could be mistaken for a heat disorder, and the bodhisattva pulse beat could be mistaken for a cold disorder.

SEASONAL PULSES

The seasonal pulses are described in terms of the conjunction of the external four seasons and the internal five elements.[29] The five elements — wood, fire, earth, iron, and water — produce certain types of pulse beats during specific seasons.

As explained earlier, the four seasons are spring, summer, autumn, and winter which are each composed of seventy-two days; the fifth season is composed of four periods of eighteen days between the seasons, again making seventy-two days. Roughly speaking, spring is the first three months of the Tibetan calendar [which according to the "Western" calendar begins at mid-winter, or around the second week of February]. The spring equinox occurs in the very middle of the season — on the fifteenth day of the second month of spring [rather than at the beginning of spring as in the "West"].

During the seventy-two days of spring, the element wood is predominant. External factors show that the season has begun, such as that the buds on trees become active, certain flowers bloom, three types of constellations appear in the sky, and larks appear. Because of the seasonal characteristics of spring, the constitutional pulses — male, female, and bodhisattva — change. In spring, the wood element is predominant, and consequently there is a strong liver pulse beat, and thus there is a tendency for the entire pulse to be subtle and taut.

Basically, everything — both animate and inanimate — has the same material basis, the five elements. Because of the cold characteristic of winter, the elements of both the external environment and internal animate beings are as if frozen. In spring a process of melting or loosening takes place; consequently, the woods — including flowers and plants — become active and bloom. A similar reaction takes place in the body; the liver has been congested during the winter, and then in spring it becomes more active. One reason why the liver corresponds to the wood constituent is in terms of its function, for just as water is channelized through the parts of a tree, so the liver channelizes the blood flow in the body.

During the eighteen day transition periods between the seasons, the earth element predominates, and since the spleen is associated with the earth element, spleenic characteristics are present in the pulse. The physician must be aware of these seasonal changes in the pulse in order not to mistake them for disease.

The fourth, fifth and sixth months of the Tibetan calendar constitute summer. Again, the major part of the season is the seventy-two days, and the remaining eighteen are the "in-between season"; the summer solstice occurs in the very middle of the season — on the fifteenth day of the second month of summer [rather than at the beginning of summer as in the "West"]. During this season, three particular constellations appear in the sky, and the cuckoo makes its song. During summer, the fire or heat element is predominant externally in the form of the heat of summer, and consequently the heart pulse beat is prominent since it corresponds to fire. Therefore, the general pulse beat during summer will be bulky and long in continuum. This information is important for reading the pulse of patients since the constitutional pulse has been affected by the season. The change is felt under all of the fingers of the doctor, not just the part reading the heart. In this sense, the topic of the seasonal pulses is an extension of the constitutional pulse section.

The seventh, eighth, and ninth months of the Tibetan calendar constitute autumn. With autumn, the constellations change; sparrows become more present and active, and plants and flowers reach their peak as fruits ripen. The iron element is predominant externally, and consequently the lung pulse beat, which is short and rough, affects the general pulse. The autumn equinox occurs in the very middle of the season — on the fifteenth day of the second month of autumn [rather than at the beginning of autumn as in the "West"].

The tenth, eleventh, and twelfth months of the Tibetan calendar constitute winter; the winter solstice occurs in the very middle of the season — on the fifteenth day of the second month of winter. In winter, the black deer begins to howl because it cannot drink from frozen lakes, and changes in the constellations occur. The water element is predominant externally, and consequently the kidney pulse beat, which is slow and gentle, is prominent since it corresponds to water. The general pulse beat during winter is affected in this way.

Mother, Child, Friend, And Enemy Pulses
As an aid to understanding the mother-child and friend-enemy relationships, the five elements — wood, fire, earth, iron, and water — are pictorialized in a vertical and horizontal manner.

		wood		
		fire		
fire	water	earth	wood	iron
		iron		
		water		

In the series of the five elements — wood, fire, earth, iron, and water — the latter arise from the former, and thus the former elements are the "mothers" of the latter in the list of five. Starting from the last element or from the bottom of the diagram, the mother of water is iron, the mother of iron is earth, the mother of earth is fire, the mother of fire is wood, and the mother of wood is water. This is the mother cycle.

Similarly, because the former elements give birth to or produce the latter, the latter are the children of the former. Starting from the beginning of the list or from the top of the diagram, the child of wood is fire; the child of fire is earth;

the child of earth is iron; the child of iron is water, and the child of water is wood. This is the child cycle.

There are also enemy and friend cycles. Starting from the left side of the diagram, the enemy of fire is water; the enemy of water is earth; the enemy of earth is wood; the enemy of wood is iron, and the enemy of iron is fire. Similarly, starting from the right side of the diagram, the friend of iron is wood, the friend of wood is earth, the friend of earth is water, the friend of water is fire, and the friend of fire is iron.

With respect to the purpose of these relationships, each vital and reservoir organ is associated with an element. The relationships are:

heart and small intestine — fire
spleen and stomach — earth
left kidney and seminal vesicle — water
lung and large intestine — iron
liver and gall bladder — wood
right kidney and bladder — water.

As explained earlier, the five elements pervade every aspect of physical experience; therefore, the condition of the elements as they change under seasonal influences is reflected internally. During spring, the wood element is most influential since the sap is flowing, twigs are budding, and so forth, and thus the pulse of the liver, associated with wood, becomes most active; that is to say, the general pulse is more influenced by the wood element and, therefore, by the liver pulse during spring and hence becomes taut and fast. The mother of liver/wood is water. Water is associated with the kidney and bladder and thus, utilizing the mother-child rule in conjunction with the seasonal pulse, if the kidney pulse in the spring has the same characteristics as the liver/wood pulse which is associated with spring, i.e., if the kidney pulse is subtle and taut, this is a sign that the patient will be successful.

If during spring the pulse of the friend of wood — the earth element and thus the spleen — is also found to be subtle and taut, the patient will have many friends during the upcoming year. The child of wood/liver is fire which is associated with the heart; thus, if the heart pulse is similar to the liver pulse, subtle and taut, in the spring, the person will become powerful and influential. The enemy of wood/liver is iron which is associated with the lungs; thus, if the lung pulse is found to be subtle and taut in the spring, the patient will face antagonism during the next year.

The same procedure is to be applied to the other seasons.

SEVEN WONDROUS PULSES

In a healthy person, pulse can be used as a means of divination.[30] There are seven types of pulse in this category:

1 family pulse
2 guest pulse
3 enemy pulse
4 friend pulse
5 evil spirit pulse
6 substitutional pulse
7 pregnancy pulse.

Family Pulse
The senior-most member of the family is examined to determine the situation of the family. The overall quality of the radial artery pulse on both arms of the patient is examined. If the pulse is sinking and as if covered over, then defilement will occur; there will be quarrels within the clan, problems with physical or emotional health, or problems with clear decision-making.

If the pulse of the senior family member is like the bite of a toothless dog, that is, very unclear, then sorrow and tragedy, such as encountering an enemy or the sudden death of a family member, will strike. If the pulse is strong and swift like a river flowing from higher land, a family member will experience extreme fright and terror. If the pulse is such that it seems to pierce the fingers, the family will experience unwanted sufferings without escape. If the pulse is similar to a hot spring, the family will become an object of gossip and defamation. If the pulse is similar to tongues of fire, that is, uneven in number and strength, there will be loss of wealth. To counteract these unfavorable indications, the physician advises the family to have certain religious rites conducted. If, however, the pulse is not faulty but accords with the individual characteristics of the usual pulse, then the family will have good fortune.

Seasonal pulse as well as the mother-child and friend-enemy cycles affect interpretation of the family pulse. If in the spring when the liver pulse is prominent, any of the six defective family pulses is present, the consequences will be experienced by the head of the family. If in the spring the liver pulse is not defective but the mother pulse — the kidney pulse — is defective, then the mother of the person having the pulse interpreted or the spiritual leader of the family will suffer. If in the spring the child pulse, that is, the fire pulse or heart organ is adversely affected, then the children of the head of the family will experience some variety of suffering. Spring is associated with wood and thus the liver, and the enemy of this complex is the lungs/ iron. If in the spring the friend, or spleen, pulse is adversely affected with one of the defective six family pulses, the wealth of the family will be affected. If in the spring the enemy, or lung, pulse is adversely affected with one of the defective six family pulses, the enemy of the family will be the one to suffer.

Guest Pulse

The guest pulse is used to determine the location of a guest who is about to visit the family. The physician examines the pulse of the person within the family to whom the guest is closest. If the liver pulse of the person being examined is strong, the guest is still at home, yet to begin his or her journey. If the lung pulse is strong, the journey is in progress. If the heart pulse is strong, the guest is close to arrival. If the spleen pulse is strong, there is a delay along the way, and if the kidney pulse is strong, an enemy or accident is encountered during the journey.

The mother-child relationship is used to determine the guest's proximity to arrival. For instance, in spring if the mother pulse — that is, the kidney pulse which is mother to the liver pulse — beats in a full manner, this indicates that the guest is still at home, etc.

In general, in regard to the seven pulses it is best to concentrate on the vital organs — the upper division pulses — as these are directly associated with the seasons.

Enemy Pulse
The enemy pulse is used prognostically by the physician to inform a person of the consequences of attacking an enemy. For example, if the attacking party has a strong lung and kidney pulse, the enemy will be conquered. If the spleen pulse is particularly strong, the enemy will be victorious. If the enemy attacks you, the opposite applies.

Friend Pulse
Here, the pulse of the head of the family is examined. If the liver pulse is strong, the family will have many friends and much wealth and will be free from unsuccessful ventures. If the heart and spleen pulses are weak and the kidney pulse is strong, the family will lack friends, will not have as much wealth, and will meet many unsuccessful ventures. If the lung pulse is strong, there will be a moderate amount of wealth and a moderate number of friends.

The mother-child and friend-enemy relationships yield further information in this context. If the friend pulse is strong, the person will be befriended by many and will accumulate much wealth. If the enemy pulse is prominent, the friend will be robbed by the enemy — others will disturb the friendship so that friends are few. If the mother pulse is prominent, then friends and wealth will be in moderation, and if the child pulse is prominent, no one will befriend the person in question. This is just a rough explanation.

Evil Spirit Pulse

Evil spirit pulses are to be taken on a healthy person whose life-situation has been affected in an unusual manner. The major characteristics of the evil spirit pulse are that it is fluctuating and changing, uncertain with sudden changes which are disproportionate to the circumstances. If the wood/liver pulse suddenly stops and is constricted and then relaxed, a mischievous evil spirit or king evil spirit is responsible. If the fire/heart pulse is affected, a fierce evil spirit and a demon, together or separate, are responsible. If the iron/lung pulse beat is affected, the king spirit and spirit caretaker of religious property, together or separate, are responsible. If the earth/spleen pulse beat is affected, an earth-owner evil spirit and *ma mo*, together or separate, are responsible. If the water/kidney pulse is affected, the trouble-maker is to be identified as a serpent spirit, a serpent vermin spirit,[31] or gnome spirit.[32]

The interrelationship of the elements through the mother-child laws and friend-enemy laws also apply to evil spirit pulses. If the mother pulse is affected, the god that is attracted and attached to the family wealth is responsible. If the child pulse is affected (for example, fire/heart in spring), the spirit responsible is the family deity of the aunt or uncle from the mother's side.

If the enemy pulse is affected (for example, in the spring if the spleen pulse is affected), misfortune is due to witchcraft. If the friend pulse is affected, then the problems are caused by spirits associated with the wealth of the family, especially those attached to certain types of wealth such as cattle, jewelry, or land. If the season pulse itself is affected, misfortune is attributed to spirits attached to the wealth of the wife or a close friend.

Please keep in mind that I am giving only abbreviated versions of these topics.

Substitutional Pulses
This pulse is used to determine the condition of a loved one or family member when the patient is unable to see the doctor. For example, in mountainous areas of Tibet a severely ill patient is often unable to travel to see a physician, but by using the pulse of a substitute person from within the family a prognosis can be made and treatment can be prescribed. For instance, if the father is ill, the pulse of a healthy son is examined. If the liver pulse of the son is complete, the father will not die, but if the liver pulse is not complete, the father will die. Mother-child and friend-enemy relationships can also be used. For example, if during spring the mother pulse of the son — the water/kidney pulse — is complete, the father will recover.

If the son is ill, it is possible to examine the healthy father. If the pulse of the heart is complete, the son will recover, but if it is not complete, the son definitely will die. In the interrelationship system, if the child pulse — the child of fire/heart is earth/spleen — is complete, recovery will occur, but if it is not complete, the disease will be fatal.

Such similarly can be applied to mother and daughter and also to husband and wife. For example, when the husband is ill, the pulse of the wife, if she is healthy, can be examined. If her liver pulse is complete, the husband will recover, but if it is incomplete, the husband will die. If the wife is sick, the healthy husband's pulse can be examined. If his kidney pulse is complete, she will recover, etc.

Through reading a substitutional pulse the character of the disorder cannot be ascertained and thus a diagnosis cannot be made. However, whether the disorder will be fatal or not can be determined, and in this sense a prognosis can be made.

Pregnancy Pulse
Pregnancy can be determined by examining the kidney

pulse in a female. If a woman is pregnant, the pulse will be protruding and rolling. If the right kidney pulse is strong, a son will be born; if the left kidney pulse is strong, a daughter will be born.

Related pulses also can be used to determine whether the delivery will be difficult or not, how easy or hard it will be to raise the child, whether the child will be prosperous, continue the family line, etc.

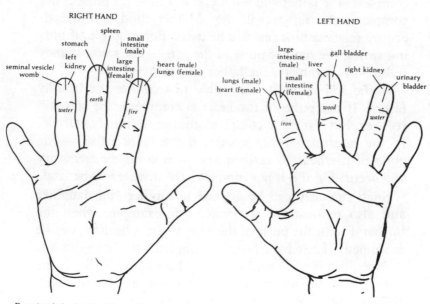

Doctor's right hand reading left arm of patient.

Doctor's left hand reading right arm of patient.

Fig. 4 Doctor's hands showing the fingertip locations used to read the various organs (see page 78-9).

8 Pulse 2

HEALTHY AND UNHEALTHY PULSES

The ninth of the thirteen sections on pulse diagnosis is one of the most important; it describes how to distinguish healthy and unhealthy pulses.[33] First, before physicians attempt to see if a person is healthy or unhealthy through pulse, they must have information as to what constitutional pulse the person has. When new patients come to the doctor, the doctor first asks them their constitutional pulse. Very often the patients themselves are aware of the importance of this information and, when they come to a new physician, immediately relate the type of constitutional pulse they have — male, female, or bodhisattva.

Out of a hundred people, the constitutional pulse location of one or two may be elsewhere on the wrist. Apart from that, in certain cases the radial artery does not yield correct information about the organs in the body. In such cases you would not use the radial artery, but this is very rare, one in a hundred or a thousand. If you are not aware of these, you could confuse the death pulse and a patient's constitutional pulse.

The first criterion in determining whether a person is healthy or diseased is the number of pulse beats that he or she has during one respiratory cycle of the physician. The physician, therefore, must follow the dietary and behavior patterns mentioned earlier and must remain calm and relaxed. A respiratory cycle involves inhaling, exhaling, and a small period inbetween the two. If the pulse rate is five times per cycle in an examination that lasts for about one hundred cycles and the beats are neither declining nor violent nor loose, etc., but regular — meaning that under each of the divisions of the fingertips the beat is of a similar type — it is definite that this person is healthy. The beats under all the fingertips must be similar; they should not vary under the index finger as compared to the ring finger, for instance. Discrepancy of beat is reason to believe that the person is not totally healthy. For instance, if under the index finger you notice a declining beat — one that seems to be slightly strong when it is first felt but slowly drops down in its inner strength — this is a sign of illness. A violent pulse beat is such that though seemingly unnoticeable, it suddenly has a strong upthrust. If you find any irregular types of beating under any of the fingertips or even under any subdivisions of the fingertips, there is reason to believe that the person is not totally healthy even within the context of the patient's having five beats per cycle.

Irregular beats that are either declining, violent, slow, quick, and so forth indicate that the person has a disorder. In terms of rate, if during one respiratory cycle the number of beats is more than five, the person has a hot disorder. If it is less than five, the person has a cold disorder.

If in one respiratory cycle there are six beats, it is a minor hot disorder. If there are seven, it is a moderate hot disorder. Eight and above indicate a severe or major hot disorder.

Similarly, if in one respiratory cycle the pulse rate is four, it is a minor cold disorder. If it is three, it is a moderate cold disorder. Finally, if it is less than three, it is a very severe cold disorder, usually incurable. The latter is described as a cold disorder that has gone beyond; that means it has gone beyond the reaches of treatment.

The requirement of five beats in one respiratory cycle which is the basis of determining health is subject to variation due to the constitutional pulse a person has. For instance, persons may have a constitutional pulse that is quick and subtle in which case the physician cannot exactly apply this standard of five beats to determine whether they are healthy or not. This means that unless the physician knows the patient's constitutional pulse, he or she could easily mistake a male or female constitutional pulse for a hot disorder or mistake a bodhisattva constitutional pulse, which is slow and gentle, for a cold disorder. Therefore, one must know whether, for instance, a bile constitutional pulse beat is inherent in a person, due to which he or she has by nature a quick and subtle pulse beat whereby the requirement of five beats in one respiratory cycle will not exactly apply. Thus, just because persons have a quick pulse beat does not mean that they have a hot disorder; they could be in perfect health.

Question: Are young children examined the same way?
Answer: No, the blood vessels in the ear are examined, as a substitute for the radial artery.

Question: Do you take your own pulse when you are sick?
Answer: Of course. It is very easy for a physician to diagnose his own illnesses since he knows very well what he has been eating over the past several days and what the qualities of those foods are, and he knows his behavior patterns and their influence on the body.

Question: Would it be possible to be phlegmic by nature and have a male pulse beat?
Answer: A person inherently predominated by phlegm can have any of the three constitutional pulses; similarly with bile and wind.

Question: Since it would not necessarily be revealed by reading the pulse, how does one determine which of the three humors predominates in a person by nature?

Answer: Pulse is most important in determining the humor that naturally predominates, but physical observation of the person is also very revealing. For instance, a person predominated by wind tends to bend one way or another whether moving about or sitting still, tends to be unable to bear the cold, to be thin, to be of darkish complexion, to be finicky about food, and, when moving, tends to give off sounds, and tends to talk a lot. A wind person is very changeable. For a conclusive diagnosis, pulse and urine must be examined but only when the patient is healthy.

GENERAL AND SPECIFIC PULSES

The tenth section is concerned with general and specific pulse beats.[34] The discussion of general pulses is in two categories: the six general hot pulses and the six general cold pulses.

The six hot pulses are: strong, expanded, rolling, quick, tight, and hard. These six hot pulses are to be viewed in terms of the three levels of hot disorders — minor, moderate, and chronic hot disorders.

If when you examine the pulse of a patient you find that the beats are numerous and superficial (superficial means that it can immediately be felt when your fingertips touch the skin on top of the radial artery), the hot disorder is a minor, or onset, hot disorder and could indicate an infection with fever disturbance. If the beats are quick and deep, it means that the hot disorder is old, chronic.

The six general cold pulse beats are: weak, sunken, declining, slow, loose, and hollow. Any of these types indicate a cold disorder. When you find that the pulse beats are deep and weak, this confirms that the cold disorder is minor or onset, whereas if you find that they are superficial (that is, when as soon as you touch the skin you feel the beats), this confirms that it is old and chronic.

The examination of specific pulse beats, by which one determines what specific disease is present, can be done in two ways. First, one examines the pulse on a common level, that is, under all the fingertips. The second method is to study it under specific fingertips, that is, in terms of each of the twelve organs represented by the two subdivisions of the three main fingertips of both hands.

With respect to the first method, studying the common pulse beat under all the fingers without considering the specific representation of the organs, the text explains that the wind pulse beat is floating, empty, and sometimes halts. It is very much like a balloon, for when you press it, you feel a depression. Here, you find a beating pulse, but when you apply pressure, the beat stops from time to time. Thus, when you notice a superficial pulse beat which, when you press it, stops from time to time and then promptly returns upon release of the pressure, that signifies a wind pulse beat.

A bile pulse is thin and taut. The phlegm pulse beat is sunken and declining.

The pulse of someone with a wind-heat [fever] disorder, also called a wind-bile disorder, is empty and quick. A phlegm-bile beat is weak on the surface, but taut deep down. A phlegm-wind pulse beat is empty and slow. The slowness indicates a phlegm disorder; the emptiness denotes a wind disorder.

In the case of brown phlegm — a triple disorder where all the three humors have been disturbed — the pulse beat will be thick, and under the middle finger you will notice a limping quality whereas under the other two fingers the pulse is weak. In a blood disorder the pulse protrudes and is rolling and superficial; it has a strong upthrust. A disorder of yellow fluid [lymph] accumulation can be determined from a pulse of a quivering nature that can also be hesitating. In case of worms being present in the body, the pulse beat will be sometimes knotty and sometimes flat. The leprosy pulse beat is limping and quivering, as if shivering.

"Limping" means that at the end it contracts like a person limping.

In the case of a fever that comes from disturbance of the body, the pulse beat is bulky, expanded, protruding, and rolling. In cases of fever that spreads to other parts of the body, the pulse is thin, hard, and tight. An infectious fever pulse is thin and quick. In cases of severe inflammation or a malignant disorder, the pulse is knotty and could be as if there are two pulse beats occurring at one time. In the case of severe pain, the pulse is short with an upthrust.

In cases of compounded [i.e., manufactured] poisoning, the pulse is strong with a short upthrust that suddenly is no longer evident. A food poisoning pulse beat is thin, quick, and limping.

An unripened, or new, fever pulse beat is thin, quick, and fluctuating; it can easily be confused with the wind pulse. A developed fever pulse beat is strong and taut. An empty fever pulse is empty, that is, when you apply pressure, the beat suddenly stops but rapidly returns when the pressure is released. A hidden fever pulse is misleading in that it has a superficial beat that seems to denote a cold disorder, but when you apply pressure deeply, you find a taut beat. An old or chronic fever pulse is thin and taut. A complex fever pulse is thin and quick under deep palpitation.

The pulse beat of wounds with inflammation or sores is bulky, hard, and quick. If gunshot or other foreign material still resides in the body, the pulse beat is limping and double, as if there were two arteries. If the head has sustained trauma of the flesh, bone, or brain such as being hit with a stone, a tight and quick pulse beat is felt respectively under different fingers. If the flesh of the head is harmed, the beat under the index fingertip will be tight and quick. If the bones of the head have been harmed, those same characteristics will be evident under the middle finger. If the brain has been harmed, a tight and quick pulse beat will be found under the ring finger.

In cases of abscess formation, the pulse has a quivering or double beat with a hot touch.

With regard to specific cold pulses, if a cold disorder is caused by indigestion and is new, the pulse beat is thick or hard. If the indigestion is of the chronic type, the pulse beat is weak and thin.

All tumor pulse beats are weak and limping. In all cases of dropsy — all three stages — it is thin on the surface but tight deep down.

If a patient vomits frequently, the pulse will be weak under the upper divisions of fingertips representing the vital organs. Frequent diarrhea will be denoted under each of the lower subdivisions representing the reservoir organs.

Possible Confusion
There are mainly six types of pulse beats from among those given above which are easily mistaken because of their similarity with other pulse beats. These are in three groups of two. First, there is great danger of mistaking a blood disorder pulse for a wind pulse. One can distinguish these, however, by applying pressure and seeing if it halts. If it does, you can confirm that it is a wind pulse beat. If it does not and continues to have an upthrust, it is a blood disorder.

The second type of confusion is between a developing fever [a fever at the point of development] and an empty fever [a fever when it is about to finish] because they are both rapid. These can be distinguished by carefully noticing that in the case of a developing fever the pulse beat is very strong whereas in the case of an empty fever it is weaker.

The third type of confusion is between phlegm and chronic blood disorders because both of these have a sunken pulse. One can distinguish them through knowing that phlegm by nature has a sunken characteristic and thus has the natural characteristics of a phlegmic pulse — weak, sunken, declining, slow, loose, and hollow — whereas such is not the case with a chronic blood disorder. In the latter case, you generally find that at the superficial level there will be a sunken beat, but when you apply pressure and feel the pulse deep down, you notice a stronger beat due to the basic prominence of the blood disorder pulse beat.

When a disorder is present, you have to determine the organ that has been affected or, in broader terms, which part of the body has been affected. This can be done by knowing that if you find defective pulse beats denoting the particular type of disorder under the fingertips of the index fingers, for instance, you can determine that the organs represented by that finger, which are heart and lungs and small and large intestines, have been affected. Similarly, the middle fingers read the liver, gall bladder, stomach, and spleen, and the ring fingers read the kidneys, bladder, and sexual organs. Generally speaking, the index fingers read the upper part of the body; the middle fingers read the middle body, and the ring fingers read the lower body.

When you read pulse in terms of the organs, you have to think in terms of the two types of pulses: the hot pulse and the cold pulse. The hot is represented by the sun, and the cold, by the moon. The hot or solar pulse is associated with the vital organs, these being known by the upper divisions of each finger, and the cold or lunar pulse with the reservoir organs, under the lower divisions of each fingertip.

In terms of what types of disorders, hot and cold, can occur simultaneously, if a hot disorder occurs in any of the vital organs such as the heart or lungs, it is possible for a cold disorder simultaneously to occur in the reservoir organs such as the stomach or intestines.[35] However, if a hot disorder occurs in the reservoir organs such as the stomach or intestines, it is not possible for a cold disorder simultaneously to affect the vital organs such as the liver or kidneys.

In terms of the location of the disease, it is possible for a cold disorder to occur in the lower part of the body simultaneously with a hot disorder in the upper part of the body. However, it is not possible for a hot disorder to occur in the lower part of the body simultaneously with a cold disorder in the upper part of the body.

Physicians have to know these points and examine patients carefully with all of their skill.

Question: How does one recognize the qualities in a subtle pulse beat? What do doctors do to keep their fingers sensitive?

Answer: You should try to keep your fingertips and hands as smooth as possible in their natural form. You should not do any type of activity whereby the skin on the fingertips becomes rough — for instance, washing a lot in hot water or working a great deal with earth or stones or touching hot metal. These affect the thickness of the skin, make it rough, and hamper sensation.

DEATH PULSES

The eleventh subdivision in the explanation of pulse is the death pulse; it is taken in order to determine when a patient will die.[36] The death pulse is calculated on the basis of (1) change, (2) incompleteness, and (3) a pause or halting in the pulse beat.

Change In Pulse

First we will consider change in the pulse beat. When a fatal disease mainly is caused by wind, the death pulse — one that indicates death — has a vibrating quality, like a flapping flag. If the disease from which the patient is to die is mainly bile and blood, the vibration is like that of a vulture's wing. If the disease is mainly of phlegm, it is like the dripping of water.

The death pulse beat of a person who has a double disorder of wind and bile is like a fish darting up to eat a fly. If the person is to die of a double disorder of phlegm and wind, the pulse is like that of a bird eating worms. If the beat is like the jumping of a frog — a frog jumps a couple of times, stops, jumps a few times, and then stops — this is a case of a death pulse of a person with a phlegm and bile disorder. If the pulse is like that of the swinging trunk of an elephant, this death pulse is of a person who has a triple disorder of wind, bile, and phlegm, involving lymph.

In the situation of a strong person who experiences a sudden trauma, the pulse uncharacteristically is of a thin and weak nature. Or, it could be that a person has had a bad disease over a long period of time and the physical constituents have been consumed and exhausted but the person has a very strong pulse. These are both signs that the person will die soon.

Similarly, if a person has a cold disorder but has the characteristics of the pulse of a heat disorder, this again is a pulse indicating impending death. The same is true if a person has a heat disorder and has the pulse beat of a cold disorder.

If in the cases of four particular diseases a patient has a normal pulse as if without disease, this again is a sign of imminent death. The four diseases are of the lungs such as in tuberculosis, food poisoning from meat, bile disorders such as in severe jaundice, and stomach disorders that are combinations of phlegm and bile.

Incomplete Pulse

Certain physical signs together with particular pulses also indicate impending death. If the heart pulse is absent and the tongue has turned black and the eyes are in a fixed gaze, the patient will die in one day. If the lung pulse is absent and the two sides of the nose shrink and the hairs inside the nose rise up, the person will die in two days. If the liver pulse is absent and the eyes rise up and the eyelashes turn inside, death will occur in three days. If the spleen pulse is absent and the lower lip sags and the sternum curves inward, the patient will die in five days. If the kidney pulse is absent and the whirring sound in the ears stops and the ears stick back to the head, the person will die in eight days.

Pauses In Pulse

The next topic is pauses that indicate impending death. One type of pause comes from illness, and another from spirits. If the pause, or arresting, of the pulse is due to an illness, the pulse of the particular organ will be affected, for it depends on what organ is diseased — whether the lungs, liver, intestines, kidneys, and so forth; the pulses of other organs will not be affected.

With regard to pauses caused by a spirit, however, there is no definiteness as to what organ will be affected. For, sometimes the pulse on one side will be hard; sometimes, on the other; sometimes it will be strong, sometimes gentle, and so forth. However, if the pause is of a regular nature — for instance, pausing at the end of every third or fourth beat, etc. — it is a sign of imminent death.

Irregular pulses and pauses also can be due merely to the influences of certain diseases and thus do not indicate impending death. Therefore, it is necessary for a physician to take great care in interpretation.

With regard to treatment, if the pause is due to spirits, various religious rites can be done to expel the spirit. If the pause is due to an illness, medicines are given to counteract the illness, but if the treatment taken for the illness is not effective, the pause in the pulse can be interpreted as indicating imminent death.

There are cases where the disease is so strong that the pulse has gone deep; this should not be confused with the death pulse. There are also cases of pulses being obscured by spirits. One has to be aware of these possibilities, for these conditions can be cured.

SPIRIT PULSES

In the case of spirit pulses, the beats are uneven in the sense that sometimes they appear on the right side or left side, or are associated sometimes with the upper body and then

with the lower body, or in terms of which organ is affected
— sometimes one and then another — or whether a hot or
cold type of pulse is shown.[37] The pulse changes suddenly
and frequently. The number is indefinite, sometimes pausing, sometimes jerky, and sometimes double.

If the spirit has affected the heart, the spirit is the god-
protector spirit[38] or king spirit.[39] If it is with the lungs, it is
a serpent spirit[40] or violent spirit.[41] If this kind of pulse is
associated with the liver pulse, it is the earth-owner spirit[42]
or ghost spirit[43] which those who have died sometimes
become.

If the spirit pulse is associated with the spleen, it is due to
a fierce earth-owner spirit or a mischievous ghost spirit.[44] If
a spirit pulse is associated with the right kidney, it is due to
a serpent and an evil spirit.[45] If it is with the left kidney, it
is a lake spirit called Tso-men[46] and an evil female serpent
spirit.[47]

In brief, if the pulse is bulky, prolonged, and unclear and
is a right side spirit pulse, it should be identified as a male
spirit pulse. If the pulse is subtle, short, and unclear and is
a left side spirit pulse, it should be identified as a female
spirit pulse. In another way, the king spirit that is the
custodian of property[48] is responsible for spirit-created
wind disorders. Violent spirits[49] and violent evil serpent
spirits[50] are responsible for spirit-created pulmonary in-
flammations. Female spirits called ma-mo-jang-men[51] are
responsible for spirit-created infectious bile disorders. Mischievous serpent spirits[52] and earth-owner spirits[53] together
are responsible for spirit-created dropsy, tumors, gout,
ulcerous growths, lupus, and leprosy.

Even though spirits cannot be seen, they definitely do
exist and bring harm. For instance, there are people with a
sore on the arm that becomes very inflamed and no matter
how much the doctor treats it, it does not heal. This would
be due to an action (*karma*) earlier in that lifetime itself, say,
in which the child harmed spirits that have taken the
appearance of frogs or snakes or if the child disturbed lakes,

forests, or ground where certain spirits reside. From doing that, the spirit comes in this very lifetime to harm. Such also can occur due to actions in a past life. Also, there are cases in which the force of one's own merit becomes used up and if a spirit in the vicinity happens to be in a strong state, it can come in and take one over. Sometimes, there are spirits who, although they are not purposely seeking to harm, like and are attracted to that being and bring harm by getting involved with that person.

Once physicians have identified the spirits that are involved, they suggest remedies such as the conduct of rituals, giving food offerings, having rites of exorcism performed by competent lamas, receiving blessings, making donations to religious persons, gaining merit through giving to the destitute, and so forth.

Question: Are such occurrences frequent, and if so, are the religious practices to get rid of them effective?
Answer: There are many occurrences; I could not even count the number of people who have been affected by spirits. The doctor has to determine the type of spirit that is causing the trouble. Then, the patient goes to the lama, monk, nun, or tantric practitioner in whom he or she has faith and asks them to conduct certain rites. When that is done, medicine given can be effective. Otherwise, no matter how much medicine is given, it cannot be effective.

Question: How can one use up one's merit?
Answer: This means using up the virtuous force of mind — the capacities established by previous good activities — and the dominance of forces established by non-virtuous actions. In order to have good capacity, you have to be able to distinguish between what is good and what is bad, and you have to believe in the cause and effect of actions. Everything done with an attitude of helping others and so forth is virtuous; actions done with opposite attitudes are non-virtuous. For instance, a person generates a very bad atti-

tude, thinking "I will kill somebody," etc.; this generates an evil frame of mind. Then the person engages in the means to carry it out — sticking a knife into the person, poisoning, etc. — and brings the action to a successful conclusion. That action will cause the person to be reborn in a hell in the future and will in this lifetime cause much suffering. Virtuous actions, for instance, are to make offferings to the Three Jewels, helping poverty-stricken sentient beings, or helping somebody who is about to die. As a result of these, one will have good companions and will be reborn in a good transmigration. These topics are very complicated and difficult.

Question: Does everyone have a death pulse all the time? *Answer*: No, if these pulses occur, they indicate that within a certain number of days you will die. Also, if the preparation for reading the pulse and so forth is done carefully, it is possible to determine if a person will die within three, four, or five years or several months, etc. Beyond that, there are other signs; if the character of the person changes in the sense that a person begins doing things he or she would not do before, this is a sign that the person will die within a few years.

LIFE SPAN PULSE

Human life is difficult to gain and is very precious once it has been gained.[54] In general, life is the basis of warmth and consciousness, as Vasubandhu's *Treasury of Knowledge*[55] says. The life span pulse is taken on the ulnar artery on the patient's wrist. If the ulnar life pulse beats normally, the life span will be normal. If it is unstable, the quality of life will be unstable. If the life pulse is nearly absent, life will end, but it can be prolonged through prayer and ritual. If the life pulse is completely absent, there is no chance for continued long life.

If the life pulse of a person who has left the household and become a monk or nun does not beat from beneath the tendons of the wrist, the protective deities of the person have changed into devils. For a layperson, this indicates a curse or manifestation of an evil spirit.

If the right ulnar life pulse in a male is as if bound and halting in character, a male relative of the patient, such as the father, will die soon. If the left ulnar life pulse in a male is as if bound and halting, the life of his wife or child will be cut short soon. If in a male both right and left life pulses are as if bound and halting, death by violence such as by being stabbed may be expected.

In a female patient, if the right hand life pulse is as if bound and halting, the husband or a relative on his side will die soon; if the left life pulse is as if bound and halting, the father or a relative on the father's side will die soon. If both the right and left life pulses of a female are as if bound and halting, her husband or children will die soon.

If either of the life pulses beats in an empty or fainting manner, loss of wealth will occur. If it is not halting but momentarily is as if bound, there will be altercations with others. If it cannot stay in its own location but shifts about, an evil spirit is present. In addition, a prominent and disturbed pulse is indicative of a male spirit being present whereas a short, coarse pulse is indicative of a female spirit.

Each beat of the life pulse in a single series that is entirely free from disorder, even, and regular reflects one year of life. Thus, a hundred such beats indicates a lifespan of a hundred years; fifty indicates a life span of fifty years, etc.

Conclusion
Pulse reveals the natures of illnesses, be they physical, emotional, or spiritual. Those who have full understanding of pulse will become famous physicians, able to serve their patients effectively. There is much more detail than what I have indicated here.

9 Questioning

The last trunk on the diagnosis root is the questioning trunk. It has three branches — questions about wind, bile, and phlegm. The branch concerned with wind diseases has eleven leaves. The first is comprised of questions about the conditions — diet and behavior — giving rise to a wind disease; for instance, the doctor asks the patient, "Have you been drinking strong tea? Have you been eating goat's meat? Have you been eating pork? Have you been doing a fast? Have you been eating food that is light and rough?" In terms of behavior, the doctor asks, "Have you been staying in a place where there are cool breezes?" Questioning about these conditions comprises the first leaf.

The next nine leaves are concerned with whether the patient has symptoms of a wind disorder. The doctor asks the patient, "Have you been yawning frequently? Have you been shaking?" Those two are one leaf. "Have you felt that you have had to stretch a lot lately?" That is one leaf. "Have you had cold shivers frequently?" That is one leaf. "Have you been having aches in hips, backbone, or in your bones in general or in your joints?" That is one leaf. "Have you had pain that is indefinite as to its location, sometimes here, sometimes there, a pain that moves around?" That is

one leaf. Then, "Have you had dry heaves?" Another leaf.
"Have you had a dulling of the sense organs?" This is one
leaf. "Have you been restless? Has your mind been such
that it cannot stay on anything, but is flying about to this
and that? Has your character been rough?" That is one leaf.
And, "Have you had more pain than usual when you are
hungry?" These are the nine leaves of questions about
whether the patient has symptoms of a wind sickness.

The last leaf is that of remedies of wind disorders — what
is beneficial in countering the disease. These are, in terms
of food, to eat oily or highly nutritious food and, in terms of
behavior, to stay in a warm place. Thus, there are eleven
leaves — one with regard to conditions, one with regard to
remedies, and nine inbetween about symptoms of the sickness itself. The first ten are questions, and the last is the
doctor's advice for curing the illness.

The second branch, questioning about a bile disorder,
has seven leaves. First, you ask questions about possible
causal conditions within diet and behavior — such as,
"Have you drunk strong beer? Have you drunk old beer?
Have you been drinking liquor? Have you been sitting a lot
in the sun or in a hot place? Have you been eating sharp and
hot foods?" These questions comprise one leaf, with regard
to the causal conditions of a bile disorder.

Due to these causes one might have become sick, symptoms of illness itself being probed by the next set of questions. "Do you have a bitter taste in your mouth no matter
what you eat? Do you have frequent headaches? Do you
have a sense of excessive heat throughout your flesh? Do
you have aches in the upper part of your body (anywhere
from the waistline up)? Do you have pain when digesting
food?" Each of those is a leaf, and thus there are five leaves
for symptoms of a bile sickness.

With respect to the remedy leaf, the patient should eat
cool food as well as bitter food, and the patient's behavior
should be cool — such as staying in a cool grove or any
place where there are cool breezes and wearing lighter

clothing.

Thus, there is one leaf about the causal conditions, five leaves about symptoms, and one leaf for the remedies. Six are questions, and the seventh is the doctor's advice to the patient.

With regard to the phlegm questioning branch, the first leaf is a set of questions about the conditions; the middle nine leaves are questions about symptoms, and the last leaf is the remedies. The first is to ask if the patient has been eating fatty meat such as that of a marmot, which is mainly fat and thus very oily and heavy. Also, "Have you eaten corn that was cooked before it was fully ripe? Have you eaten various types of beans or peas that were not fully ripe?" In terms of behavior or conduct, "Have you been sitting or lying down in a wet area?"

With respect to symptoms of a phlegm sickness, "Have you had a loss of appetite, such that you do not feel to eat anything? Has your stomach inflated upward [heartburn]? Has a sour taste tended to rise in the mouth? Belching frequently? Have you had heaviness of body and mind such that you do not feel to move your body or do not feel to involve your mind in anything? No matter what you eat is it difficult to digest? Frequently vomiting? No matter what you eat do you have no sense of taste of that food — you can't taste whether it is sweet, sour, or whatever? You're cold in body outside and inside? You're cold right from inside your body and you're cold outside on the surface too? As soon as food arrives in the stomach, you have pain, a sense of sickness?"

In terms of remedies, the patient should eat food that is light, warm, and rough and that is easy to digest. In terms of conduct, one should stay in warm places.

Thus with regard to phlegm there is one leaf of questioning the patient about causes that promote phlegm disorders, nine with regard to symptoms, and one leaf of remedies.

Question: Are the symptom leaves in an order indicating

increasing severity?
Answer: It is not that as you go down the leaves the illness
becomes more severe. These are signs of these respective
illnesses themselves. When there is a double or triple disorder, the symptoms of the three illnesses become mixed in
one person.

Question: To have one of these diseases do you have to have
all of the symptoms of the particular humoral sickness or a
majority of them?
Answer: If, for instance, a phlegm disease is particularly
severe, you would have all of them.

Question: Are the symptoms listed here the only symptoms
for each of these disorders?
Answer: There are more; these are just a general compen-
dium. With regard to wind, for instance, there also are
increases of wind and great increases of wind as well as
losses and great losses of the potency of wind. There are
different categories of increase, exhaustion, and disturbance of the particular humor. Thus, the lists are general
categories.

There are thirty-eight leaves on the diagnosis root
altogether. The observation trunk has two branches —
tongue observation and urine observation with three leaves
each. The pulse feeling trunk has three branches and
three leaves. The questioning trunk has three branches and
twenty-nine leaves — eleven, seven, and eleven. Through
knowing these signs you can definitely identify a patient's
illness.

Question: Have the number of leaves been the same for
centuries, or have certain leaves been added on? In the next
century will there be forty leaves?
Answer: This is a general description in accordance with the
basic nature of humans, but there are differences with
regard to the number of *diseases* in certain centuries. For
instance, Shākyamuni Buddha predicted the arising of

various diseases in later times.

Question: Is there a type of mental questioning for the bile branch such as that for wind when the physician asks about mental roughness and for phlegm asks about heaviness of mind?
Answer: No. There is none for bile. Most types of mental illness arise from wind problems. The fluctuation of the mind is due to the nature of wind which is light and fluctuating.

Question: Can diseases caused by actions of a former lifetime be told from these methods of diagnosis, such as by checking the pulse or urine?
Answer: It is very difficult to tell when a disease is caused by an action in a former lifetime. Since I am not a special person, such as a Bodhisattva who might be able to tell immediately upon seeing a person, I do it by going through a process of diagnosis, administering medicine, and then seeing if the medicine helps or not. Determining whether a disease is due to an action of a former lifetime is a process of inference. It cannot be known directly by someone like me.

Question: What about genetic inheritance? Can families all be predisposed to wind, etc.?
Answer: No. Even the shapes of the faces of children of the same parents are not the same. Similarly, their dispositions as to what they like to do, eat, think, what pleases them, and so forth, are not the same. These are due to former actions in a previous lifetime. Such topics are extremely complex; for instance, that a stupid child is born to stupid parents might mean that the child had done an action in common with those two persons in a past lifetime and that it has caused rebirth in this situation. A person such as I am cannot speak about these complex matters.

Question: What about preventive diet? If someone is basi-

cally a wind person, would a preventive diet help?
Answer: For people who have wind, bile, or phlegm predominance naturally and are not ill, these same remedies are helpful.

Question: What is cool food?
Answer: Salad and cabbage are cool. Even if you cook cabbage and eat it hot, it is still a food with a cool potency. Cooking it makes it a little lighter, not so heavy.

Question: What about spices?
Answer: Spices could make the dish become warmer, for instance.

Question: Do problems with pregnancy or menstrual disorders come under any of these categories?
Answer: There are some forty strictly female disorders, involving any of the humors — wind, bile, phlegm, and blood — but they are mostly wind and blood problems. There are separate explanations of these in the medical literature.

Question: Can you give examples of hot and rough foods?
Answer: Grains that are grown in dry areas. Hot pepper. Anything that has a hot taste. Here in this country you do not eat many hot foods; you mostly eat sweet foods, it appears.

Question: If you are, say, predominantly a wind person, would you be more prone to wind disorders?
Answer: Yes, but I cannot say that a person whose nature is wind would necessarily have more wind disorders, and it is the same with the other two humors. The frequency of illness depends upon factors of food, conduct, and so forth at the particular time.

Question: Do you see a predominance of these types in different age groups?

Answer: Yes. The predominance of wind, bile, and phlegm comes about in three ways — the person's nature, the person's age, and the person's locality. Adults have a predominance of bile. The aged have a predominance of wind. Children have a predominance of phlegm. In terms of locality, in high places persons have a predominance of wind; in low places that are dry and hot, bile; and in oily or damp places, phlegm. If an old person is staying in a place that is cold and the person is, by nature, of the wind type, the physician has to prescribe the ultimate wind medicines because of the unfavorable combination. Thus, when doctors give medicine, they must consider factors of locality, season, age, and nature.

10 Urinalysis

Just as one looks into a mirror and sees an image, so does a qualified physician look into a patient's urine and from this see the disorders of the patient.

The discussion of urinalysis has many parts: preparation for urinalysis, the proper time for such observation, the vessel or cup in which the urine is placed for diagnosis, and the manner in which the coloration changes due to passing through the various organs.[56] Also, there are four general types of urinalysis: of ordinary persons without any major illness, of persons with disorders, of persons on the verge of death, and of persons affected by spirits. Thus, altogether there are eight general subtopics.

PREPARATION FOR URINALYSIS

If a patient's urine is to be diagnosed in the morning, then the night before there are certain types of behavior that should be followed. One should avoid any strong tea as well as very much yogurt or any beer or alcohol. The reason for this is that taking any of those substances affects the coloring and so forth of the urine, making it difficult for diagnosis.

Furthermore, during the night preceding urine diagnosis

one should not go without liquid altogether, such that the following morning one is extremely thirsty. In other words, just be normal, take sufficient liquids so you are not terribly thirsty. One should not have sexual intercourse the night prior to diagnosis. Nor should one stay awake at night; get a good night's sleep.

One should also not go to excess in moving about or in trying to stay in just one position. Nor should one allow a great deal of tension or a great deal of thinking. Do not go to any excess prior to diagnosis.

With respect to the urine to be diagnosed, it should not be that from urinating during the time before four or five in the morning; since urination at such a time is affected strongly by the food taken the previous meal, it is not good for diagnosis. One should use the urine that builds up in the hours around four or five in the morning. If one does not urinate during the night, then do not collect the first half of the urination when you rise; use only the later half.

TIME FOR URINALYSIS

There are three aspects of urinalysis: color, vapor arising from the urine, and the albumin which is a cloud-like substance in the urine. The time for such diagnosis is after dawn.

THE VESSEL

The vessel in which the urine is to be placed is most often a white porcelain cup which is such that its color will not affect the appearance of the color of the urine. Otherwise, an aluminum pot can be used. One should not use vessels that color the urine, such as a clay, copper, brass, or any other colored pot; they make the urine appear to have another color, and it will be difficult to tell what the natural color of the urine is.

A white cup is best and not one with a pattern in it. If it is impossible to get one of these three appropriate types, one can line another type with a piece of white paper.

COLORATION CHANGES

With respect to variations in the urine, the fourth topic, the text speaks first of the digestive process. In the stomach, food is differentiated or separated into a nutritious or more subtle part and a less nutritious or unrefined part. The refined or better part goes to the blood. The more waste-like product goes to the intestines. In the intestines it is divided in two, that is, into solid and liquid parts. The liquid portion of this waste goes from the intestines to the urinary bladder.

With regard to the separation in the stomach, the finer or more nutritious part goes to the liver. Within this, there is another separation between the more nutritious and the less, with the more nutritious part becoming blood and the less nutritious going to the gall bladder. In the gall bladder there is a further separation, the finer substance becoming lymph. The more wasteful part becomes albumin, the cloud-like substance which appears in the urine; the albumin goes together with the urine and accumulates in the urinary bladder. It is because of this separation in the process of digestion that food which has been ingested affects or transforms the color of the urine.

The albumin, or cloud-like substance, basically appears in urine due to blood and bile problems. Therefore, the condition of the body in terms of heat and cold is indicated in the urine. Just as in the marketplace when a merchant has something illegal to sell and does not actually reveal it, holding it under a garment, describing it and from that you can tell what he has hidden, so from the urine it is possible to tell the types of disorders or lack thereof in a person's body.

THE URINE OF HEALTHY PERSONS

If one looks at the urine of a healthy person, one finds that its color is more or less the bright, cheerful yellow of the butter on top of the milk from a "dri", the female counterpart of the yak [yaks only being males]. The odor is like that of the cream that rises to the surface of milk. The vapor is neither terribly strong or weak, neither big or small, and the duration of the vapor — before the urine gets cooler and the vapor stops — is neither terribly long or short. The bubbles or froth are nothing spectacular — neither terribly long or short, big or small, rather moderate froth on top of the urine.

The albumin, for a healthy person, is simply mixed up together with the urine, pervading it. Also, for a healthy person there is not much chyle (the oily substance normally rising to the surface of the urine); just a little bit comes to the surface. As the vapor gradually vanishes, one finds that a little darker color converges toward the center of the cup of urine, just as breath on a mirror gradually converges in the center and disappears. After the urine has cooled off, its color is light, clear, and yellowish; it is transparent.

THE URINE OF DISEASED PERSONS

Concerning the urine of persons with disorders, there are two aspects to the discussion: general and specific diseased urine.

GENERAL URINALYSIS

There are three times for diagnosing the urine: when it is hot, then when it is lukewarm, and finally when it is completely cooled off.

There are nine types of diagnosis that are broken down into three groups relative to the three times. First, when the urine is hot, one checks the color, the vapor, the odor, and the type of bubbles or froth. When it is lukewarm, one checks the cloud-like albumin and the oily chyle that rises to the top. When the urine is cooled off completely, one checks the time of the variation of the color, then how it changes, and finally postponed analysis. When patients are not able to come themselves, their urine is sent, in Tibet by yak, in India by other means. It is rather old by the time it arrives, and so the doctor checks everything, but with a different type of diagnosis, because the urine is older. This is called "postponed analysis".

Urinalysis When the Urine is Fresh
Color. We return to the first of the nine, the color, which is investigated when the urine is still quite hot. The urine of a person with a wind ailment is like water from a mountain spring, light blue in color and transparent. A bile disorder will manifest in the urine as a more yellow, perhaps even an orangish, color. If the urine is very pale, or whitish, this indicates a phlegm disorder.

Question: Is there a difference between the blueness of the urine of a wind disorder and the paleness of a phlegm disorder?
Answer: The urine of a person with a phlegm disorder is a bit milky as if someone took milk and dropped it into the urine; you cannot see through it. For the wind disorder it is very clear, like mountain spring water.

If the urine is red, it indicates a blood disorder. If the urine is rust color, this indicates a lymph disorder. If the urine is brownish, it indicates a complex disorder of all three humors — wind, bile, and phlegm.

If the color is a mixture of red and yellow, it indicates a disorder of blood and bile. If it is a mixture of white and yellow, this indicates a disorder of both phlegm and bile. If the urine is yellow, like mustard oil, and oily, it indicates both a bile disorder and contagious disease.

If it is orange, thick, and has a foul odor, this indicates a type of disorder that spreads from organ to organ or a general disturbance of the body, such as with a heat ailment. If the color of the urine is generally dark but has a spectrum of color, like a rainbow, this indicates poisoning; it could be any variety of poisoning — mineral, meat, and so on.

Vapor. The second of the nine types of diagnosis is vapor, which is investigated while the urine is very hot. If the urine has a large vapor, this indicates a developed heat ailment. If there is little vapor but it lasts a long time, this indicates either a hidden heat ailment or an old, chronic heat ailment. If there is little vapor that lasts a short time, it is a cold ailment, involving phlegm and wind — an excess of cold in the body. If there is an alternation in the amount of vapor, then in that case there exists a combination of heat and cold disorders in the body.

The vapor is seen just as, for example, you see steam rise from a cup of hot tea. Bubbles, color, and vapor are visual.

Odor. The odor of the urine is, of course, to be smelled. If the urine has a foul odor and there is albumin in the urine, this indicates a strong heat disorder. If there is either no odor or a very slight odor, this indicates a cold disorder. If the urine smells of different foods such as cabbage, meat, and so forth, this indicates that the digestion is not working properly; the digestive heat is not up to par.

Froth. If the froth or bubbles on the urine have a bluish tint and are large, this indicates a wind disorder. If the bubbles are small and many and, when stirred, pop quickly, it indicates a bile disorder. If the bubbles remain static on the surface of the urine like the bubbles of saliva, as if you spit into water, this indicates a phlegm disorder. If the bubbles have a reddish tint, this indicates a blood disorder. If they are varicolored like a rainbow, this indicates poisoning. If they form in the cup and then very quickly disband like a flock of pigeons or doves who are dive-bombed by a hawk and go off in all directions, this indicates an old disorder which now pervades the body; it has become serious.

Four points have been described for urinalysis while the urine is still hot: color, vapor, smell, and froth.

Urinalysis When the Urine is Lukewarm

Albumin. When the urine has become lukewarm, one analyzes the albumin and the oily chyle. The albumin or cloud-like substance in the urine appears, for the most part, only in cases of heat disorders — illnesses of blood and bile. If, when the albumin forms in lukewarm urine, it is very subtle, like a hair on the arm, this indicates a disorder of the wind. If the albumin forms on the surface like the wool-like film on the edge of a stream, this indicates a disorder of blood and bile.

If the albumin forms subtly on the surface of the urine, like the white tips of the hairs of a rabbit, and you almost have to squint to see it, this indicates a phlegm and cold disorder. If the albumin forms like a cloudbank pervading the urine, this indicates a lung disorder such as tuberculosis. If the albumin is like pus, this indicates that there is probably an infection or pus in the body, possibly in the stomach or kidneys. If the albumin congeals on the surface in little grains like sand, this indicates a disorder of the kidneys.

Remember that when albumin appears in the urine, it usually indicates a heat disorder, as it basically arises from bile and heat. If the albumin appears on the surface, this indicates a heat disorder of an organ in the upper part of the body, specifically the heart or lungs. If the albumin appears in the bottom of the urine, it indicates a disorder of the kidneys. If it is in the middle, it indicates a disorder of either the spleen or the liver. If the albumin pervades the urine, this indicates that the physical constituents as well as the heat/cold factors of the body have been disturbed, agitated by the winds.

Concerning the thickness of the albumin, if it is quite thick, this indicates a heat disorder. If it is very thin, this indicates a cold disorder, though, as mentioned above, the presence of albumin generally indicates a heat disorder.

The color of the albumin will be that of the urine of the particular person at that time. For example, a bile disorder will make the albumin orange. Or, for example, if the urine itself were like rainbow color from poisoning, the albumin would likewise be of different colors.

Chyle. If the chyle — which, being an oily substance, always comes to the surface of the urine — is thin, this indicates a cold disorder. If it is quite thick, it indicates a heat disorder.

Sometimes the oily chyle is quite thick, becoming noticeable when the urine sits for fifteen or twenty-four hours, gradually congealing at the surface, like butter on Tibetan tea. If it is quite substantial, the doctor can delicately take it off the surface of the urine with a thin instrument. Then he puts a few drops of it on a hot red coal, and if its smell is like that of barley or other grains when heated, this indicates that there is a disorder that will cease by itself and thus does not need to be treated.

If the oily chyle forms on the surface in crisscrossing bands, this indicates a tumorous growth, not necessarily cancerous. This phenomenon occurs for all types of tumors. Subsequent analysis will reveal what type of growth it is.

There are also times when a spirit or malignant being, a non-human being, can be recognized from this oily substance when it forms certain patterns or shapes on the surface of the urine. This is just mentioned in passing, to be discussed in detail later on.

This completes the second major section, the diagnosis to be done while the urine is lukewarm.

Urinalysis When the Urine is Cold
Now, we come to the third section, diagnoses done mainly when the urine is cold; it has three parts — the time of the variation of the color, how it changes, and the postponed analysis.

Time of the variation of the color. If, when fresh hot urine is poured into a cup, the color changes rapidly before the vapor has even vanished, this indicates a very strong heat ailment. Vapor occurs at the time of urination itself when it is naturally hot; normally, when it is brought to a physician, it has already gotten cold, so the vapor would already have passed, and it does not rise again if the doctor takes it from a jar and pours it into a cup. Thus, this particular diagnosis is not relevant after the urine is cold even though it is set forth in this section; it is done before the vapor is gone. To repeat, at the point of urination the urine is quite hot, then as it cools down, the vapors stop coming up. If during this period the color is already changing, that indicates a heat disorder.

Question: Should the patient report this to the doctor?
Answer: No, this is too much to expect of the patient. Sometimes the doctor will go to the patient's house and check it.

If the color of the urine changes after the vapor has already vanished and the urine has cooled, this indicates a cold disorder. If the color changes as the vapor vanishes, this indicates a balance of the heat and cold elements of the body; thus, there is neither a heat nor a cold disorder. There might be a disorder, but not of these types because the two are in balance.

How the color of the urine changes. If the color of the urine gradually congeals in the sense that the darker coloration gathers in the center of the cup, this indicates a cold disorder. If you see that the color changes from the depths of the urine, rising up together with the albumin, this indicates a new heat disorder.

If you find that this darker coloration of the urine converges towards the center in rims or rows non-homogenously, this indicates an old heat disorder. If the color of the albumin changes before the color of the urine, this indicates a disturbance or conflict of the heat/cold elements of the body, or a heat disorder that now pervades the body, or a cold disorder now come to fulfillment — that is, it might start out in the kidneys and move on to the other constituents, until it affects all of them.

If there is a disorder caused by a spirit or if a person is on the verge of death, the urine of the patient does not change — the color is constant.

Postponed analysis. The last topic is called delayed or postponed analysis — this being conducted after the analyses mentioned above. This type of investigation can be done, for instance, even when the urine has come from a long distance, and so it could be even several days old, not just freshly cold. In such a case, the color of the urine will correspond to the color of the basis of the disorder — wind, bile, or phlegm; for instance, with a bile disorder the urine will be orangish. If the urine is quite dense, it is a heat ailment. If it is watery or very fluid, this indicates a cold disorder.

SPECIFIC URINALYSIS

Having finished the general presentation of urinalysis, we move to the specific analysis, about which there are two parts: discusssions in terms of heat and cold ailments.

When a heat disorder is present, the urine will be either red or yellow, and it will tend to be rather thick with a foul odor and have a great deal of vapor which lasts a long time. The bubbles that rise to the surface will be small, many, and quickly vanish, and the oily chyle that rises to the surface will be in a thick layer. The albumin — the cloud-like substance — will pervade the entire urine, tending to converge towards the center of the vessel.

Furthermore, in the case of a heat ailment, before the warmth of the urine dissipates and before the vapor has stopped rising, the color of the urine is already changing. When the urine is completely cooled down, the color turns dark, or brownish, and the urine has become thick, dense.

With regard to the qualities of urine in the case of a cold

disorder, the color will be very pale or bluish. It will be very fluid rather than dense. Both the vapor arising from it and the odor are slight — not much of either. The bubbles are large in size. The oily chyle and the albumin both just form a thin layer; there is very little of either. The color of the urine changes only after the heat and the vapor have passed. When finally the urine is completely cooled down, it takes on a bluish tint and becomes a thin liquid.

With regard to the type of urine in cases when there are combinations of both heat and cold disorders, there could be, for example, a heat disorder in the inner part of the body while on the surface there could be a cold disorder, or in different parts of the body there could be disorders of both of these elements simultaneously. In these cases, the color of the urine may be pale with a bluish tint, and there could be a thick layer of the albumin, the cloud-like substance. If such signs are apparent, this indicates a slight cold disorder but essentially or deep down a serious heat disorder. Such a condition can be quite deceptive; that is, one looks at the urine and by the color thinks there is a cold disorder, but by the thick layer of the albumin you know there is also a heat disorder. It is easy to misdiagnose the patient in such a situation.

Another example of such mixture is when the color of the urine is orangish, but there is little chyle and no albumin. In such a situation it would appear that there is a heat disorder, but in fact far more serious and more predominant is a cold disorder as can be known from the paucity of albumin and chyle.

Again, earlier it was said that in the case of a heat disorder the color changes quite quickly. However, if the color change occurs much later or if a urine basically seems to indicate a cold disorder but, instead of changing slowly, changes color quite quickly, in both of these two cases a hidden heat disorder is indicated. In the first case, the urine basically indicates a heat disorder, but one sees that the color changes slowly. In the second case, a basically cold disorder urine changes in color quite quickly. Both of these indicate a hidden or concealed heat disorder. Again, this can be quite deceptive; there is danger that the physician might misdiagnose the illness.

With urine that is analyzed as essentially indicating a heat disorder, if one finds that there are no bubbles, this indicates that the heat disorder has sunk down into the abdominal region; it has gone quite deep into the body. On the other hand, if the urine basically suggests a cold disorder but there are no bubbles, this indicates that the cold disorder has become chronic.

If the urine basically suggests a heat disorder and there is a thick layer of oily chyle, the physical constituents (nutritional essence, blood, flesh, fat, bone, marrow, and regenerative fluid) are dissolving. The physical constituents are being lost, as a result of which one becomes anemic, in very poor health, weak.

If the urine indicates a cold disorder, but one finds oily chyle in the urine, this indicates that with the cold disorder there is a problem in digestion such that one is not digesting butter, oils, and fats.

In general, it is possible to confuse heat disorders which involve the winds. A combination of a heat/wind disorder which has become chronic can be mistaken for a heat disorder combined with blood. Another that is easily confused is a disorder of all three of the basic humors — phlegm, bile, and wind — for it can be mistaken for a lymph disorder, such as rheumatism. The former can be confused on the basis of color, the red of the urine, and the latter can be confused on the basis of the brownish color of the urine.

It is possible to confuse disorders in the kidneys, liver, and spleen because disorders in these organs all result in red urine. It is easy to confuse these three disorders.

When the urine has a bluish tint, it is possible to confuse a hidden heat disorder and a cold disorder involving an imbalance of both phlegm and wind. Both of these result in urine with a bluish tint, making it possible to confuse one for the other.

The preceding have been warnings, general statements that it is easy to confuse this for this, etc. In conclusion, the text admonishes the reader to be careful, not to confuse them, to identify properly all characteristics of the urine of each disorder by studying larger and more involved commentaries.

THE URINE OF PERSONS ON THE VERGE OF DEATH

We move on to another major category, that is, the urine of persons who are on the verge of death. With regard to the characteristics of such urine, first of all, if the color is red like blood and has a rotten odor like rotten leather and if, despite the physician's prescribing certain medication, behavior, or diet, the patient does not improve and the odor of the urine becomes stronger and stronger, this indicates that the person will die, specifically of a heat disorder.

If the albumin, the cloud-like substance, remains static in the urine, without changing, the person will die. Also, if the urine has a bluish tint, no odor, no vapor, and no taste and if treatment has no beneficial effect, this indicates death as a result of a cold disorder.

If the urine has many lines in it — little patterns — and it has a bluish tint, this indicates death as a result of a wind disorder. The lines are like those on the surface of the water when you boil spinach. If the urine has these same lines or patterns and has a yellow or orange color, this indicates death as a result of a bile disorder. Still, when the urine has these same lines in it and the color is reddish, this indicates death as a result of a blood disorder. If the urine is like old, curdled milk and has these lines in it, this indicates death as a result of a phlegm disorder. In each of these cases one should realize that there are strata in the urine, with different colors and so forth.

The next one is, again with these lines in it, like pouring

black ink into water and then letting it separate. Thus, if the color is blackish, this indicates death as a result of poisoning.

If there is water accumulation in the abdomen but without kidney disorder, this indicates death as a result of a disorder of all three humors.

URINE OF PERSONS AFFECTED BY SPIRITS

The eighth and last section on urinalysis deals with the diagnosis of malignant spirits that harm persons. The patient takes a large vessel, places it on a low table, and without picking it up urinates into it. The direction of the vessel from which the patient urinates will simply be called east. The physician leaves it overnight without touching it, during which time patterns emerge. A grid, like the lines on the back of a turtle, is used as a tool of analysis to determine what type of entity is harming the patient. (See charts on following pages.)

Malignant Spirit Urinalysis For A Male Patient

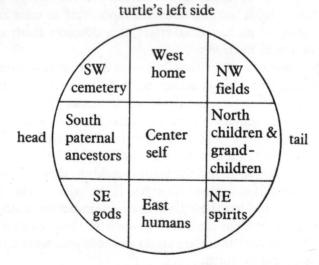

turtle's left side

turtle's right side

For a male patient

The turtle lying on its back

E — right side of the turtle
S — head of the turtle
N — tail of the turtle
W — left side of the turtle

Locations Of Harming Spirits

SE — gods
E — humans
NE — spirits
SW — cemetery
W — home
NW — fields
S — paternal ancestors
Center — oneself
N — children and grandchildren

Malignant Spirit Urinalysis For A Female Patient

turtle's right side

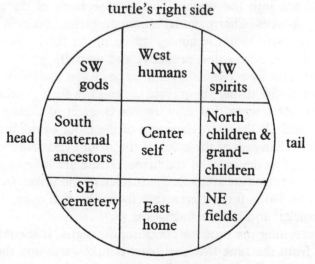

turtle's left side

For a female patient

The turtle upright
E — left side of the turtle
S — head of the turtle
N — tail of the turtle
W — right side of the turtle

Locations Of Harming Spirits
SW — gods
W   — humans
NW — spirits
SE — cemetery
E   — home
NE — fields
S   — maternal ancestors
Center — oneself
N   — children and grandchildren

This grid is placed over the surface of the urine as you look down into the vessel. The nine sections of the grid signify sources of harm: gods, humans, spirits, spirits in the cemetery, spirits in the home, spirits in the fields outside, ancestors on both sides, progeny, and oneself.

With this as a basic diagram or grid for analyzing the surface of the urine, the physician watches for (1) various patterns or images that may appear in each of these nine places and (2) the swift changing of the color of the urine, the slow changing of the color of the urine, and sometimes no change in the color of the urine. These are investigated for each of the nine areas on the surface of the urine. In the grid, one looks for patterns that look like fish eyes, lines like cracks, and bubble formation.

Concerning the time for checking the signs, it should be done from the time that the urine is lukewarm and thereafter as the urine becomes completely cold. More often than not the doctor will not have the opportunity to check the urine when it is still lukewarm; he will have to do it when it has already cooled.

It is important not to bump the vessel. If the doctor disturbs the urine in any way, it makes the whole process useless; he must leave it just as it is. The bubbles and patterns form naturally. He mentally superimposes the grid on it and performs the diagnosis in the above fashion.

First of all, in terms of the actual diagnosis, if one finds that the square relating to "gods" is different whereas all the others are homogeneous in their bubble formation and so forth, this indicates that there is harm inflicted by a god and specifically one with whom oneself or one's relatives have had a relationship that has gone awry. For instance, perhaps one was showing devotion and making propitiation for some time to that "god" and then stopped. In any case, something went wrong, and disturbance in this square indicates harm at the hands of such a figure.

If special signs occur in the square relating to human beings, this indicates harm inflicted by a human spirit, simply, a ghost, called a scent-cater. If special patterns occur in the square related to spirits, it is specifically harm inflicted by the chief spirit of the world when this world first formed. When a world forms, there arises a predominant spirit with it; this is what is indicated here.

If the special indications occur in the square relating to one's ancestors, this indicates harm by a spirit that comes about in one of two ways: (1) a person has acquired a certain possession, usually a precious or expensive one, which certain spirits cling to such that they harm the people owning it or (2) a spirit has been incited to harm an individual by a sorcerer who has such ability.

If the special indications occur in the square relating to progeny, it suggests harm inflicted by a spirit from one of one's aunts or uncles, on either side of the family. I will not explain all of the indications; the above is sufficient to illustrate the type of diagnosis that is done. For each of the sectors, specific spirits are indicated, and there are descriptions of types of spirits in terms of the direction of the grid that has been affected and the specific form of the patterns that appear. Such detail is not needed for our purposes here.

The layout of the grid as given above is for a male. For a female it is reversed; the turtle is turned over so that it is right side up, no longer on its back as it was for a male. Thus, except for the center sections, all the other sections are reversed.

In conclusion, it is said that urine is like a mirror. Just as a mirror reflects images, so urine reflects all diseases.

TONGUE OBSERVATION

With respect to the observation trunk on the diagnosis root, it remains to describe how the tongue looks in diseases of wind, bile, and phlegm. Briefly, the tongue in a wind disorder is red and a little dry with many small bumps around the edge. The tongue in a bile disorder is covered with a yellow coating; the patient has a bitter taste in the mouth. The tongue in a phlegm disorder is covered with a gray and sticky coating.

In a brief and rough way, this concludes discussion of diagnosis. Now let us turn to treatment.

PART THREE

TREATMENT

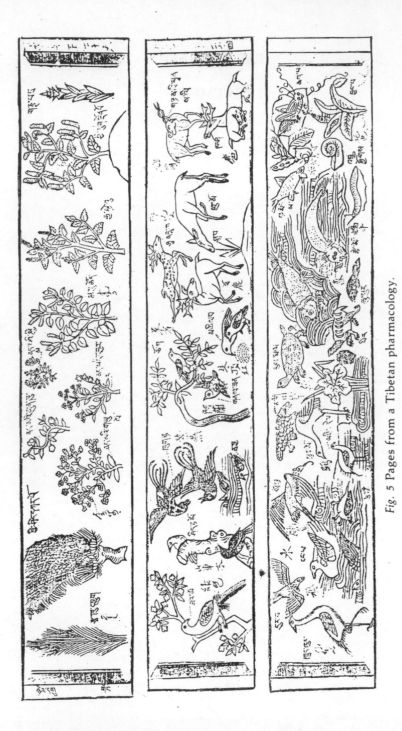

Fig. 5 Pages from a Tibetan pharmacology.

Healing Root

4 Trunks, 27 Branches, 98 Leaves

Food Trunk
(1) Wind food branch
1. Horse meat
2. Donkey meat
3. Marmot meat
4. Year-old meat
5. Meat of hero killed in battle
6. Seed oil
7. Year-old butter
8. Molasses
9. Garlic
10. Onion
(2) Wind beverage branch
1. Hot milk
2. Wine of Angelica root and Polygonatum cirrhifolium
3. Wine of molasses
4. Bone wine
(3) Bile food branch
1. Yogurt of cow and goat milk
2. Whey of cow and goat milk
3. Fresh butter
4. Meat of wild herbivorous animals
5. Goat meat
6. Fresh meat of hybrid yak-calf
7. Fresh barley porridge
8. Grey dandelion
9. Dandelion porridge
(4) Bile beverage branch
1. Boiled water
2. Cold water from rocky and snowy mountain
3. Boiled water cooled off
(5) Phlegm food branch

    1. Mutton
    2. Wild yak meat
    3. Wild carnivorous animal meat
    4. Fish
    5. Honey
    6. Aged barley and meat porridge
(6) Phlegm beverage branch
    1. Yogurt and whey of "dri" (female yak) milk
    2. Aged wine
    3. Boiled water (taken hot)

Behavior Trunk
(1) Wind behavior
    1. Staying in a dark warm place
    2. Sweet conversation with beloved friends
(2) Bile behavior
    1. Staying near sea shore or in cool breezy place
    2. Soft gentle conduct
(3) Phlegm behavior
    1. Physical exercise and exposure to sun's heat
    2. Staying in a warm place

Medicine Trunk
(1) Wind medicinal tastes
    1. Sweet: molasses
    2. Sour: aged wine, vinegar
    3. Salty: red rock salt
(2) Wind medicinal potencies
    1. Oily: black agaru tree, eaglewood
    2. Heavy: black salt
    3. Smooth: rosy leadwort
(3) Bile medicinal tastes
    1. Sweet: raisins
    2. Bitter: wild cucumber
    3. Astringent: white sandalwood
(4) Bile medicinal potencies
    1. Cool: camphor

2. Liquid: Cassia fistula
3. Bland: bamboo mannu
(5) Phlegm medicinal tastes
   1. Hot: black pepper
   2. Sour: pomegranate
   3. Astringent: Chebulic myrobalan
(6) Phlegm medicinal potencies
   1. Sharp: red rock salt
   2. Coarse: Hippophae rhamnoides (berries)
   3. Light: white leadwort
(7) Wind alleviation by soup
   1. Soup of sheep's ankle bone
   2. Soup of four essences: meat, wine, brown sugar, butter
   3. Soup of head of sheep kept for one year
(8) Wind alleviation by medicinal butter
   1. Nutmeg butter
   2. Garlic butter
   3. Three fruits butter (Chebulic myrobalan, Beleric myrobalan, Emblica officinalis)
   4. Five roots butter (Withania somnifera, wild asparagus, Polygonatum cirrhifolium, Asparagus racemosus, Black aconite)
   5. Monkshood (Black aconite) butter
(9) Bile alleviation by decoction
   1. Root of Iris germanica
   2. Heart leaved moonseed
   3. Chiretta
   4. Three fruits (Chebulic myrobalan, Beleric myrobalan, Emblica officinalis)
(10) Bile alleviation by powders
   1. Camphor
   2. White sandalwood
   3. Saffron
   4. Bamboo concretion
(11) Phlegm alleviation by pills
   1. Monkshood (Black aconite)

    2. Various salts
(12) Phlegm alleviation by powders
    1. Pomegranate
    2. Rhododendron authopogonoides
    3. Hot, i.e. pungent, medicine (a heat formula)
    4. Calcified salt
    5. Calcite
(13) Wind alleviation by suppository
    1. Suppository followed by shaking legs upwards
    2. Suppository followed by beating soles of feet
    3. Suppository followed by feet being shaken
(14) Bile alleviation by purgative
    1. General purgative
    2. Specific purgative
    3. Strong purgative
    4. Mild purgative
(15) Phlegm alleviation by emetics
    1. Strong emetic
    2. Mild emetic

Accessory Therapy Trunk
(1) Wind
    1. Hot moxabustion, hot application, anise seed
    2. Massage with sesame oil
(2) Bile
    1. Inducing perspiration by wearing heavy clothes
    2. Venesection
    3. Cold water bottle fomentation
(3) Phlegm
    1. Hot application
    2. Moxabustion

11 Behavior

Recommendations for behavior are given in three categories: continual, seasonal, and occasional behavior. The first is broken into two parts: continual behavior for the entire life and religious practice.

CONTINUAL BEHAVIOR FOR THE ENTIRE LIFE

Everyone wants happiness and a long life and does not want suffering, and everyone engages in techniques to achieve these.[57] In order to get rid of suffering — disease — and to lengthen your life span, there are various methods which you can employ. You can wear precious stones on various places of the body to lengthen your lifetime and protect from disease. You also should take medicine that accords with your own physical disposition, and you should seek the help of protector deities through the practice of Secret Mantra.

You should, with mindfulness, avoid the two conditions giving rise to illness: unsuitable eating habits and unsuitable behavior, these being, for instance, to drink mixtures of different kinds of alcoholic beverages, to stay out in the sun for a long time and then come in to the cold, to wear light clothing in the winter, and to wear heavy clothing and so forth in the summer. You also should in all ways abandon as much as possible the various forms of the non-virtues — three physical: killing, stealing, and sexual misconduct; four verbal: lying, divisive speech, harmful talk, and senseless chatter; and three mental: covetousness, harmful intent, and wrong view. You should diminish these as much as you can.

The sense faculties — the tongue sense and so forth — should be used in a balanced manner; you should, for instance, not gaze too much at the very beautiful or the very ugly or prolongedly smell very attractive or very unattractive odors. If you gaze at very ugly things too long, eventually the wind element in the body is stirred up. Similarly, if you smell bad odors too much, it eventually affects the wind element in your body, and this brings out illnesses.

You should avoid getting on a wild horse, swimming in a whirlpool, running through fire to show off your courage, climbing up and jumping down from trees in summer to show off your physical prowess, or playing at the edge of caverns that are filled with water from the rains of summer. At all times in all seasons, you should avoid such activities, basically because they could kill or harm. For instance, if you hang on branches, they could easily break off, or if you swim in a whirlpool, you can get sucked in; riding on a wild horse, you can get thrown off, injured, and even killed.

When walking, you should watch the road carefully. When staying in a single place, you should know the area where you are staying. You should try not to go about in the night, but if there is something important for which you have to go outside, take a friend along for protection. Do not go against the nature of things, in terms of time and in terms of the nature of the situation.

One reason for taking care about where you go and where you stay and so forth is that if, for instance, you go into the woods, you could fall into a trap that has been built to capture deer. If you do not watch where you are walking on a narrow bridge, for instance, when you get to the end you might fall into a trap constructed for animals — the bridge itself being part of the trap. In other words, you have to take care.

It is advisable not to fast all the time, or sleep during the day instead of the night, or put great effort into tasks at which you cannot possibly succeed. Do not get drunk from alcohol a great deal; this will cause the strength of your body to be lost. Do not stay talking all the time, just chattering on and on. These will cause your body to become old before its time.

In the spring [or late winter according to the "Western" seasons], when the nights are becoming shorter, it is a very rough season, and thus it is not a time to spend fasting, chattering, or any of the other above mentioned activities; if you do, this will cause your body to lose strength and the wind element to increase. Thus, if during this season you sleep a little bit, just after noon, it is very helpful. For instance, if you sleep for a half hour or an hour after lunch in the spring, it counteracts the effect of these activities — counters the loss of strength of body and counters the increase of the wind element.

If in the summer, fall, and winter, however, you sleep after lunch, this will cause an increase of phlegm; body and mind will become heavy, the sharpness of your intelligence will lessen, you will not want to move around much, you will get lazy, and you will get common colds over and over again.

A person who has to sleep a lot should be given an emetic and fast afterward. The purpose is to vomit out the phlegm that causes heaviness, and thus a special emetic is needed in order to expel the unwanted phlegm.

A person who cannot sleep should at noon take warm milk and at night take broth made from lean meat. The insomniac should rub sesame oil all over the top of the head. Also, in a spoon melt a little pure fresh butter and at the point at which it cools off, take just a drop and put it in each ear.

In general, you should not commit adultery, that is, lie with somebody who is married or who is under the care of another person, nor should you fornicate with animals. You also should not copulate during the time of menstruation. In the winter you can copulate as much as you wish — there is no specified limit — but in the fall and spring you should not copulate more than twice a week. In the months of summer you should copulate no more than once every two weeks. This is because summer is the peak time of the elements; since everything is highly developed, if you copulate a lot during this time, your strength will be lost.

If more copulation is done, this will cause your sense powers (eye, ears, nose, tongue, and body) to become dull. For instance, your sight will not be as clear or bright. It can also cause untimely death; if, for instance, you had been capable of living one hundred years, you might die at seventy or eighty. Also, your intelligence will become duller.

In order to overcome the wind that causes you to age, you should bathe frequently and then rub sesame oil everywhere on the body. In India we can get only sesame oil, but here you have many kinds of oil that are suitable although mustard oil is to be avoided. This will get rid of fat, and your body will be lighter. Rubbing oil on the body will increase the digestive fires; your intelligence will become clear, and you will have a clear sense of exertion. It also increases sexual powers.

Question: How often is "frequent" bathing?
Answer: It is *necessary* to bathe at least once a week, but you *should* do it twice. In India people who practice this bathe every day in the morning and then rub on oil.

Question: If you copulate more than the specified number of times, is there any counteraction you can take?
Answer: Yes, there is medicine. There is a separate text on virilification and aphrodisiacs for the sake of restoring sexual potency — making the impotent potent. It is said in that

text that if a man takes this medicine properly, he can lie with a hundred women in one night. I do not know about that, but the medicine is very powerful.

If you transgress these rules, it is possible to contract chronic disorders. These specifications of times and season and amounts are particularly important for the old, for children, and for those who have a predominance of either wind or bile. They are slightly less important for the adult who is not bothered by wind or bile problems.

Persons who have a strong body should take fatty and oily types of foods in the winter and spring. However, they should lessen the intake of these in the summer and the fall, the reason being that fatty and oily foods will increase bile.

Most important for a person who is predominated by phlegm is any form of exercise — running, jumping, swimming, whatever. When a person who is predominated by phlegm washes, as a substitute for soap, or in mixture with soap, it is good to use powdered lentil. It draws out phlegm in the hair pores. Through this, your joints will be very flexible. This also causes fat to dissolve, and the flesh to improve. If you engage in such behavior, your skin will have good tone, your limbs will be very strong, and you will have a long life.

Question: What other kinds of oil are good to use?
Answer: Oils from various types of nuts, even walnut oil, but not mustard oil.

Question: Can you bathe too much or have sex too seldom?
Answer: If you bathe many times during the day, the water itself might increase wind problems. With regard to having too little sexual activity, I do not think there would be much fault, except for the possible formation of stones.

Religious Behavior
Because all sentient beings want happiness, they engage in

many activities; in the previous section, we talked about worldly activities; now let us turn to religious activities. Because it is the case that even regular happiness can lead to suffering, it is best to engage in religious activities. You should not procrastinate with regard to religious practice, thinking that you can accumulate wealth and a good situation and then practice later on. Rather, you should begin practicing right away, not putting it off until later.

The main religious activities are: with regard to physical acts, to give up killing living beings, stealing, and impure sexual activity — adultery; with regard to verbal activities, you should give up lying, senseless talk, harmful speech, and divisive talk which is the worst of all; mentally, you should give up covetousness which is a desire to have somebody else's belongings, harmful intent which is to wish to harm another, and wrong views — for instance, to view that there is no cause and effect of actions, that there is no rebirth, that there is no such thing as Buddha, Doctrine, and the Spiritual Community. In this way you should give up non-virtuous activities — three of body, four of speech, and three of mind. Even if you are unable to sit in a cross-legged posture and have the appearance of one who is meditating, the diminishing and abandonment of these is religious practice.

Whatever capacity you have should be used to help those overwhelmed by sorrow, those bereft of wealth, and those stricken by suffering. Helping others is very special. You should always view any living being, even bugs and so forth, as like yourself. Just as you would not like a needle stuck in your own flesh, so even a worm or bug does not like such things.

You should, when talking to others, speak altruistically with a smiling face, without deception, and honestly. You should mainly seek to help even persons who are acting as your enemy and are trying to harm you. Also, with a motivation of love you should generate the two altruistic supreme minds of enlightenment — the altruistic intention to become enlightened in both its aspirational and practical forms as well as the realization of the emptiness of inherent existence.

Physically, even if now we are not Bodhisattvas and are incapable of giving our own bodies to others, we can give gifts to others; we can give blood to others who do not have enough. Persons who make organ donations are indeed carrying out the Bodhisattva precepts. *Verbally*, we should use our speech with an attitude of altruism; for instance, if another is seeking to kill someone and trying to find out where they are, even if you had seen the intended victim, you can tell the killer that you do not know where that person is and thereby free that being from being killed. Similarly, *mentally* you should think about what will be helpful to others, discriminating between what helps and what harms others.

It is very important to engage in the Bodhisattva type of altruistic attitude, considering others' welfare to be more important than your own. These are the ultimate religious practices.

Question: What happens if you feel anger but are smiling?
Answer: It would be harmful because you are angry, but because of not carrying out an action of harm against someone else, the effect would be less.

Question: It seems that you run the danger of self-deception rather than the deception of others when you attempt to act differently than you feel.
Answer: Once you have desire and hatred, there is no way that you cannot be in a position of loss. If you show it to others, it will bring a certain problem and if you keep it inside, it will bring another. We are stuck in this situation until attaining freedom from the afflictions of desire, hatred, and ignorance.

SEASONAL BEHAVIOR

With regard to behavior suited to the seasons, the year is divided into four seasons: winter, spring, summer, and autumn.[58] There are 21,000 respirations in one day. Thirty days to a month equals 630,000 in a month. Each of the four seasons has three months, making 7,560,000 respirations in a year.

The spring equinox occurs on the fifteenth day of the middle month of spring. [The beginning of the "Western" spring is the Tibetan midpoint of spring.] The fall equinox occurs on the fifteenth day of the middle month of fall. The winter solstice, the longest night, occurs on the fifteenth day of the middle month of winter. The summer solstice, the longest day, occurs on the fifteenth day of the middle month of summer. The eighteen days between each season, explained earlier for pulse reading, do not apply here.

In the middle of spring, the days are becoming longer, and the sun is moving to the north. At the time of the summer solstice the sun has gone as far to the north as it can. That is the fifteenth day of the middle month of the summer. Then it starts going to the south. A point of equal day and night occurs on the fifteenth day of the middle month of fall, the autumnal equinox. Then the sun continues going south, going farther and farther away from us; the days get shorter, and the nights, longer. The longest night, when the sun has gone as far south as it can, is the fifteenth day of the middle month of winter, the winter solstice.

Because the sun is starting to go north at this time, the elements are becoming rough, hot, and sharp. Since the strength of the sun increases from this point, these qualities increase. Then from midsummer, the summer solstice, when the sun starts going south, the cool quality of the moon increases. It is because of these factors that you have to engage in seasonal behavior.

Specifically, from the fifteenth day of the middle month of winter, the cool quality of the moon and the elements of earth and water diminish in strength, and the hot and astringent tastes of foods increase. These cause people in late winter and early spring to lose their strength and to have to eat more. Because the elements of fire and wind are increasing, your own strength naturally decreases.

At the summer solstice, because the sun starts moving to the south, the elements of earth and water begin to increase. This means that you naturally become stronger, and thus it is not necessary to eat so much during this period. This is because water and earth serve as the basis — they are firm — causing you to become stronger until the winter solstice when your strength is at its peak. Again, at the winter solstice, when the sun starts moving north, wind and fire begin to increase and thus burn up your strength.

From the middle of the summer the rainy season begins; the falling of rain causes the elements of earth and water to increase, thereby naturally increasing the potencies of sour, salty, and sweet tastes, which, in turn, increase physical strength. This is because the moon qualities increase from the summer solstice on. In the first month of winter, the last month of spring, the last month of summer, and the middle month of autumn the elements are in balance.

It is on the basis of such a division of the months of the year that the medical texts set forth modes of behavior for particular times and seasons. The first part of winter is very cold, and thus the hair pores are blocked. Since the wind in the body is as if hiding the power of the fire, if you eat only a little, your physical strength will diminish. You should eat a lot of foods strong in the tastes of sourness, saltiness, and sweetness.

Because the nights are long during this season, you become hungry, and from this viewpoint your physical constituents also diminish. For, if you get hungry during the long night, this will cause the physical constituents to decrease.

With regard to bathing, during this season you should rub on sesame oil after bathing. Also, you should eat fatty meat, oily foods, butter, and meat broth. You should put on furry clothing and cover your feet with shoes, boots, and so forth. You should expose yourself occasionally to a little heat, the heat of fire and of the sun, but be careful not to get overheated.

You should stay in houses that do not let in breezes, not in just a shack of boards. Since the twelfth month is particularly cold, you should take special care at that time with respect to these modes of behavior. [The twelfth month of the Tibetan system is the "Western" January, roughly speaking.]

During winter, phlegm accumulates in the body; because the weather is cold, the accumulated phlegm is as if freezing — becoming solid — inside the body. Then, in spring [which would roughly be February, March, and April] the light of the sun is warm, due to which the accumulated phlegm melts and, as a result, the fiery warmth of digestion degenerates; hence, phlegm diseases will rise. To keep them from rising, you should partake of the three tastes — hot, bitter, and astringent, such as hot spicy foods, hot peppers, non-oily herbs, grains left for a year — aged but not rotten — and the flesh of animals living in dry places such as mountain goat meat. Also, you should eat honey and drink water that has ginger boiled in it. All these are very helpful.

This behavior should be started a month and a half before and continue a month and a half after the spring equinox. It is a time for exercising — running, bowing down to images, etc. When you wash, you should use lentil powder instead of soap, or mixed with soap, rubbing it on the body and then washing it off. Through these activities phlegm will be cleared away. Also, put pleasant scents on your body. Stay in places where there are pleasant flowers, stay some in a pleasant grove, and stay in a partially shady place where there is sunlight coming through leaves.

Then at the end of spring and the beginning of summer, the light of the sun is hot. Due to this, the body is robbed of strength, and thus you should eat food that is sweet in taste, cool in potency, light, and oily. For instance, pork is cool and light. You should avoid salty, hot, and sour food as well as exerting yourself a lot in exercise. You should give up staying out in the sunlight; sunbathing will harm. Do not bathe with hot water; use cool water. Drink a mixture of beer or liquor and cool water, or put ice in your drink or in your beer.

Open the windows and put on screens. Wear light clothing. Put pleasant odors on yourself and in the room; this will keep bugs away, and that, in turn, will keep disease away. Since bugs come to dirty places, due to the pleasant smell bugs will not come. Burning incense is very good. Also, set out fragrant flowers. Stay in the shade of trees, in a place where the breezes will bring the pleasant odor of flowers to you.

During late summer in the rainy or monsoon season, everything is damp from the water brought by the rain. This stirs up and dirties the waters because there is a cold wind that blows when it rains. Thus, the water you drink in this season becomes worse; even if you draw it up from deep in the ground, the source of that water is still stirred up and dirty. Due to that, the digestive fires become weaker, and thus you have to use techniques to increase them. You should take foods that are sour, salty, and sweet — as in early winter — as well as food that is light, warm, and oily. Drink beer or liquor from grains grown in dry places. Avoid cool places.

Even though late summer is cool because of the rain, there is also great heat when the clouds clear, due to which you can suddenly be bothered by great heat too. The bile that has accumulated during the rainy season from eating oily food and so forth can rise during autumn as diseases; therefore, in order to clear away the bile, you should, toward the end of the third month of summer, take foods that are sweet, bitter, and astringent. The astringent does not have much taste to it, neither sweet nor sour nor salty; there are many medicines that are astringent. You should surround yourself with odors that are not only fragrant but also cool. Camphor, white sandalwood, and *ushi* wood, which is somewhat like white sandalwood, are good. These can be burned as powders in a pot and taken throughout the house, just as you should mix camphor with water and sprinkle it throughout the house after sweeping.

In brief, with respect to food, in monsoon season and winter you should take warm food. In the spring you should take rough food. In early summer and the fall, you should take cool food. In the monsoon season and winter, you should take foods that are hot, salty, and sour. In the spring, you should take the three tastes of bitter, hot, and astringent; in the fall, sweet, bitter, and astringent.

If you are naturally phlegmic in character, in spring you should take a special emetic to vomit out the phlegm. Or, if you are predominantly of bilious nature, in the fall you should take a special purgative that causes evacuation of the bile. If you are predominantly windy by nature, in late summer you should use a special enema to counteract wind.

All of these recommendations for diet and behavior should be adjusted to take account of variations from the norm within seasons, such as when it is hotter or cooler than usual. You will live longer and without disease if your behavior accords with the season.

OCCASIONAL BEHAVIOR

There are thirteen types of occasional or temporary behavior to be considered: hunger, thirst, vomiting, yawning, sneezing, breathing, sleeping, clearing mucus in the throat, expelling saliva, defecation, expelling gas, urination, and emitting semen.[59] You should not forcefully suppress any of these thirteen.

If you forcefully suppress hunger, the faults that develop are a deterioration of the body in general, physical weakness, pain in the throat after swallowing, and dizziness. For a remedy, frequently take light, oily, and warm foods.

If you suppress thirst, the faults that occur are dizziness, heart ailments, and dullness of mind — a loss of clarity. The antidotes are different types of cool foods, cool drink, and cool environment.

Not allowing yourself to vomit will lead to a loss of appetite, difficulty in breathing, a disease that involves swelling of the face and hands, sores, itchiness, sores that will not heal, leprosy, disorders of the eyes, and also a tendency to get the common cold again and again. If you come to have this disorder, the remedies are to fast, to inhale the smoke of aloewood and sandalwood, and to drink frequently small amounts of fluids such as water with honey in it.

From not allowing yourself to sneeze, the faults that will arise are a general lack of clarity of the senses, dizziness, stiffness of neck to one side, a twisting and distortion of the mouth, and also a lack of strength in the cheeks. The remedies are to inhale the smoke of aloewood and sandalwood, nasal medicine that clears the nose, and to look toward the sun.

From not allowing yourself to yawn there is not a great deal of fault. Whatever harm there is can be readily removed by taking wind medicines, engaging in activities recommended for avoiding wind disorders, and also eating food that is good for balancing wind disorders.

If you engage in severe forms of physical exertion, such that it interferes with your breathing — for example, holding something very heavy for a long time such that you cannot breathe right — or if you do not allow yourself to breathe deeply after exertion, these are very harmful, leading to various types of tumors and to heart ailments. The remedy is to rest well; medicine is not needed.

If you do not sleep when needed, this brings on a great deal of yawning, a general physical slowness — you do not feel like doing much — heaviness of the head, dimness of vision, and difficulty of digestion. The remedy is to drink meat broth, to drink beer, to rub the body with oil, and to sleep.

If you do not remove the mucus that accumulates in the throat, more mucus will accumulate, interfering with breathing, making it hard to breathe. Also, it will lead to loss of weight, a tendency to hiccups, and to heart disorders. The remedy is to get rid of the mucus in the throat through taking certain liquid medicines.

If there is excess saliva and you keep it in your mouth, this can lead to pains in the heart and the head, a runny nose, and dizziness. The remedies are to drink beer and to sleep. There is no need for medicine; if you drink beer, rest, and leave it alone, it will get better.

If you do not expel gas, this will lead to a drying of the excrement which will lead to general constipation. A further consequence can be the formation of tumors as well as pain. A long-term effect can be heart trouble.

If you frequently do not defecate when you feel the need, this can lead to a bad smell from the mouth, pain in the brain, cramps here and there in the body, and a tendency to get the common cold frequently. For this it is necessary to take a purgative.

Obstructing urination can lead to formation of stones in the bladder and the kidneys and to diseases of the urinary organs as well as the male and female sexual organs. The medicine is applied topically to the male or female organs. Also, one rubs oil on the body, applies hot or cold towels to parts of the body, and takes a medicine that is basically a vitamin.

If you obstruct the emission of semen, it can cause pain in the male organ, eventually leading to a blockage of urination, the formation of kidney stones, and impotence. The medicine for this is inserted in the sexual organ; one also soaks in medicinal baths, and intercourse is recommended. Also, you should eat sesame oil, milk, and chicken, and should drink beer.

With respect to these thirteen, you definitely should not either forcefully obstruct these thirteen or do them forcefully such as in straining while defecating. You should allow them to occur naturally, not applying force to cause or prevent them. Doing either of these disturbs the physical constituents, leading to many types of ailments. The winds are disturbed, and this throws the physical balance off. To keep such from occurring, you always should eat properly, take the proper medicine, and engage in proper types of behavior.

To purify the body from seasonal accumulations, you should take a special emetic in spring to vomit out the phlegm, accumulated during the winter, which, otherwise, will rise as a cold disorder in spring. During the monsoon season and the winter, you should take a special enema to purify the body of wind disorders that have accumulated in early summer. In the fall, take a special purgative to clear out the bile that has accumulated during the monsoon season.

As a way of preventing disorders from arising in the body, you should always engage in these modes of behavior with respect to foods, behavior patterns, and so forth. If you act in this way, the body will be balanced, and, therefore, disorders will not arise. If a disorder should arise, you should immediately tend to it — while it is still relatively minor — by adjusting your behavior.

Question: You said that for some things fasting was prescribed, but if you fast you would feel hunger, and you said that prolonged hunger is bad.
Answer: It is true that in a healthy state you should satisfy hunger, but if you have a set of symptoms, such as difficulty in breathing, loss of appetite, swelling, spots on the skin, etc., that are due to having suppressed vomiting, then it is a different situation, and you need the remedy of fasting. The remedy will not give you the symptoms of not eating because it is a different situation.

Question: How do you build the motivation to change behavior that produces humor imbalances?

Answer: Because people are very busy, they tend not to take the time to pay attention to their own health. However, if you look through the list, you will see that from suppressing some of them you even can get tumors of various sorts and that suppressing others can lead to heart and other serious disorders. By seeing that from rather small things serious consequences can arise, you should decide to be more careful.

Another difficulty is that often local customs are against not suppressing these things. For instance, it is not polite to sneeze or blow your nose or clear your throat or cough; it is considered embarrassing to expel gas in public. Such cultural prohibitions are harmful to health. Formerly, in Tibet and China, the custom was for people to keep a small spittoon made of whatever one could get — valuable or not — on a table near you; it was commonplace to spit excess mucus into it, but nowadays you must use a handkerchief, which is not as easy.

Question: Is yawning just a sign of sleepiness or does it serve another function?

Answer: Yawning is not just a sign of a need to sleep; it also indicates a wind disorder. If you have frequently prevented sleep, yawning can be a sign of tiredness, but mainly it is a sign of wind disorders. This is why the text says that to counteract having suppressed yawning, you should use remedies to wind disorders.

Question: Would deep breathing help the wind disorder?

Answer: It might help a little, but not much. Basically wind disorders, of which yawning is a symptom, are of three types: either the wind potency has increased, has diminished, or is disturbed. Deep breathing can help the type that is a disturbance. To counteract diminishment of wind, you have to eat very strong foods, high in nutritional value, and also take medicine.

Question: I have found that when I go to a place with high altitude, it takes a while to adjust. Is there anything you can do to adapt faster?

Answer: It will help to drink a little beer and not to drink coffee; it is all right to drink tea. If you cannot get beer, make a broth of lean meat bones; it will help.

12 Diet: Grains and Meats

If you partake of food and drink well, your body and life will be sustained well, whereby you will live long.[60] If you do not know how to eat and drink properly — if these are insufficient, excessive, or perverse — diseases will be produced, and your body and life will be adventitiously over-powered. Hence, those who want happpiness should value skill in eating and drinking.

The general discussion about diet is divided into two parts, food and drink. With respect to foods there are five sections, the first being on grains [including legumes], the second on meats, the next on oils, the fourth on greens, and the last on spices.

GRAINS

Among "grains" there are two types: those that are in pods and those without pods — as in the difference between peas and wheat.

Those that do not have pods are rice, millet, a red round type of grain called "tra-ma"[61] [quick "60 day" barley] which has a sharp point, wheat, barley, thick-shelled barley[62] which has a very tough husk, "say-da"[63], a green-ish type of grain which has a point that is bent like a hook whereas wheat and barley have a straight point, and so forth.

Roughly speaking, their taste is sweet and their post-digestive taste is also sweet. These foods produce virility, overcome excessive wind, generate physical strength, and increase phlegm.

Specifically, among these, rice is oily, soft, cool, and light and thus can clear away faults of all three humors — wind, bile, and phlegm — can increase virility, and stop vomiting and diarrhea. Millet is heavy and cool, thus causing the body to be stable; it also mends bones. It brings back together bones that are out of place and bones that are broken.

"Tra-ma" is cool, light, and rough. If you eat much of this, it will steal away your appetite.

Wheat is heavy and cool; it sustains the body in the sense of generating physical strength and clears away wind and bile without increasing phlegm.

Barley is heavy and cool. It increases feces and is supreme for generating strength.

Thick-shelled barley which has a very tough husk and "say-da", a greenish type of grain which has a point that is bent, are cool and light, and thus they clear away phlegm and bile.

Question: In a heavy grain diet, how can one overcome the phlegm that would build up? Is there something that one should eat with it?
Answer: You should not eat grain alone but also eat various vegetables and so forth. If you did not eat anything else with it, indeed it would increase phlegm, but not otherwise.

Legumes
With respect to podded "grains", the many varieties can be divided into two groups by way of size, big and small. They are also divided on the basis of whether the "grain" [i.e., the bean] is flat or round.

The taste of beans is astringent and sweet. Their potency

is cool, light, and non-oily; hence, they cause the channel passageways for blood, wind, and so forth to be constricted. Also, they clear away heat disorders of the phlegmic variety and eliminate diarrhea in that they constrict channels, including the passageway for feces. As was said earlier, in place of soap, one could use lentil powder to reduce phlegm. If you put such powder on your fatty areas, it will help by pulling out the fat and oil. Also, if a fat person eats a lot of podded "grains", it will help to reduce fat; it will make you thin. Thus, these podded grains get rid of oil as well as blood and bile.

A Chinese bean,[64] a reddish or whitish bean with a thick skin, not shaped like a kidney, other than being used externally as indicated above, should not be eaten frequently because it will increase phlegm-wind in the form of respiratory problems. It will cause more mucus and your breathing to be uncomfortable — it aggravates asthma. It helps hemorrhoids and diseases associated with that. It also will help to overcome the formation of semen stones, and it generates blood and bile.

"Ma-sha"[65] [soybean], which is used to make tofu and ping [bean thread], are white and a little bit like a kidney, with a design. They overcome wind and cause an increase of phlegm, bile, semen, and strength.

There is a small flat red bean[66] that you can open up into two parts [red lentil]; it increases all three humors. Its taste is astringent and sweet. It is ground into powder, and as one of its usages, it is rubbed on the body when one has a blood problem manifesting as itchy spots here and there. You make powder, mix it in a little water, and put it on those places. It is also used for a problem with the heels of the feet. If you have high blood pressure, eating it will help.

Sesame grains, both white and black,[67] are heavy and warm. They promote virility and overcome wind disorders.

Linseed, called "sar-ma"[68] in Tibetan, is small, flat, and red and is pressed for its oil. It can be powdered and cooked and can be prepared like ping. It is sweet, oily, and soft. It helps wind.

Buckwheat, called "dra-wo",[69] is of two types: white and yellow, found inside a triangular fruit. Plentiful in Tibet, Nepal, and India, they are cool and light. If you have sores with blood and pus and put a powder of this on them, it will draw out the pus. Also, eating them will clear away sores. It generates all three humors.

All of these grains and beans, whether podded or unpodded, when newly harvested and until dried over the period of a year, are heavy. Thus, their potency is heavy if you eat them right away after harvest, at which time they increase phlegm and hence are not appropriate for eating. However, if harvested when mature and if dried over a year, they are light in potency and suitable for eating. If you eat grains harvested when not fully ripe or when they have not dried for a year, you will tend to get diarrhea.

If you eat grains or beans raw, they are heavy in potency and difficult to digest, but if you eat them cooked or also mixed with other foods, they are light and more digestible. If cooked and mixed with other foods, they are even more assimilatable.

Question: If podded "grains" constrict the channels, do they constrict breathing?
Answer: If you eat a lot of these, the worst is that this will cause the winds not to circulate well. However, for someone whose wind is moving too much and is losing a lot of blood — for instance, from the nose — these would help.

Question: Does "eating a lot" mean eating the item week after week?
Answer: Even if you ate beans moderately every day, that would be all right, but eating too much too often would be harmful.

CLASSES OF ANIMALS

There are eight classes of meat from three types of animals

— those that stay in dry places, such as in the mountains; those that stay in wet places, such as in the ocean, lakes, and so forth; and those that stay in both.[70]

Birds are divided into large and small birds; the former walk whereas the latter hop. The first class of birds is comprised of those that dig in the ground for food with their claws — peacock,[71] grouse,[72] partridge,[73] jackdaw which is a black bird with a red beak called "kyung-ga",[74] and a "black bird"[75] which is similar to the former one and is frequently eaten in India.

The second class is birds that dig out food with their beaks. These are: parrot, i.e., a yellow bird with a red beak that talks;[76] cuckoo,[77] which is a white bird with a white beak that stays near water; stockdove,[78] which is a white bird like the former but has a long beak and red legs and stays near water; magpie;[79] "jöl-mo"[80] whose body is either white, red, black, or yellow, stays in trees, and has a beautiful voice; sparrow,[81] a dark-headed bird that stays near houses; other birds that go into fields and eat grains; and so forth.

The third category is wild herbivorous mammals: deer,[82] musk deer,[83] antelope[84] which have white hair at the tail with the male having horns, a type of wild sheep called "nyen"[85] which has a huge, heavy horn structure due to which it generally dies in old age, rabbit,[86] "dzö"[87] which has long narrow straight horns, burrhel sheep,[88] and so forth.

Also in the third category are larger wild herbivorous animals: "gya"[89] which is like a cow, spotted deer[90] which is smaller than the former one, wild goat,[91] wild boar,[92] water buffalo[93] which is like a yak with big horns and of which there are yellow and brown types, rhinoceros,[94] tiger that stays in bamboo groves,[95] wild ass[96] which is a horse-like animal that stays in mountains, wild yak[97] which is like the buffalo that I have seen in your movies, wild cross-breed of yak and cow[98] which is like a wild yak but with wide thick horns; and so forth.

The fourth category is carnivorous animals: tiger;[99] leopard;[100] bear;[101] yellow bear[102] which is a big animal with a large forehead that will rise up and even grab a person and tear it in half — its feet being like a human's but it does not have heels; it has a white spot on the chest and is yellow or black; snow leopard[103] which is like a leopard but has a long tail; "jang-kyi" [wolverine?][104] which is like a dog but bigger even than a wolf and which will eat sheep, yak, and even horse; lynx[105] which is a white animal with tufted ears that feeds off the blood of animals; wolf;[106] hill-dog[107] which is a little bigger than a dog, has very bright fur, and moves in packs with the animals jumping back and forth over each other; "dray"[108] which eats humans; and so forth. Hill-dogs spend all night traveling about, the one feeling that he is stronger than the others and showing off by jumping over another; it is a lot of fun to watch them cross a big river, the current of the river carries them away but they help each other by holding onto each other's legs; they will jump on the back of a horse or sheep and reach down and break into the stomach, killing them; even before the animal dies they will clear out the whole abdomen.

The fifth category is birds that eat by the power of their dexterity: vulture;[109] magpie;[110] red vulture;[111] kite[112] which is a big black bird that sweeps down on rabbits or small sheep and carries them away; crow;[113] owl;[114] sparrow hawk[115] that eats hopping birds; and so forth.

The sixth category is domesticated animals. The first is a "dzo"[116] a hybrid with a cow as the mother and a yak as the father. The female hybrid of a "dri"[117] [the female version of the yak] and your buffalo give a lot of milk, and the offspring of these hybrids — when the father is a bull — gives even more milk, but it is hard to keep alive. Still, its child gives endless milk; it is like a jewel because the milk keeps coming. You get over one hundred glasses of milk per milking from the first type of hybrid [six and a half to seven gallons]. They are very expensive; in India they cost about five thousand rupees. One of the relocated Tibetan colleges in south India has one, but the people do not know what they have and do not take care of it. The second in the list of domesticated animals is yak;[118] the male is called "yak", the female "dri"[119] — when Westerners talk about yak milk, we Tibetans laugh a lot. Next are camel;[120] horse;[121] donkey;[122] cow and bull;[123] "gom-bo"[124] which is a hybrid cow that is thin and gives a lot of milk; goat;[125] sheep;[126] dog;[127] pig;[128] chicken;[129] cat;[130] and so forth.

Most of these animals are found in Tibet; the herbivores are more prevalent in the north; the carnivores are more prevalent in the south; among birds, the larger are more prevalent in the west; and the smaller, in the east.

The seventh category is animals that live in holes. The first is marmot;[131] its flesh is extremely oily, such that if you put a piece of it in a bottle, in time oil will drip out through the bottle. It lives in holes in the ground and moves about under the ground. Next is porcupine [or porcupine-type flying squirrel?][132] which is like a bird but its feathers are needle-pointed like a pen, very sharp; if you grabbed it, its feathers would stick into you. If a dog came to grab it, its feathers or quills would stick into it. If you throw a stone at it, it will stick up its quills, whereby the stone will not hit it. It flies a little. To kill it, you throw a big radish or potato at it; it puts up its quills, and the radish or potato sticks into them, due to which the animal cannot fly.

Also in this category are toad;[133] snake;[134] badger[135] which is like a cat that lives in a hole in the ground; lizard;[136] chameleon[137] which goes in sand no matter how hot it is and changes color; scorpion;[138] and so forth.

The eighth category is animals that live in the damp: crane[139] which has long legs and a long neck; grey teal;[140] duck[141] which is yellow in color; heron[142] a big black bird that cannot go into water to get fish, so it stays on the shore and, as the waves push them up, it catches them; bittern;[143] otter[144] which is like a cat, has legs and a tail, and just eats fish; fish[145] of which there are many types; and so forth.

Meat

The flesh of the animals in all eight categories is sweet in taste and sweet in post-digestive taste; their potency is sweet. These eight [or nine when smaller and larger herbivores are separated] are divided into three groups. The first three — those that dig out food with their claws, those that dig with their beaks, and the smaller herbivores — are animals that stay where it is dry. The last two — those that live in holes and those that live in dampness — are animals that live in moist places. The middle four — bigger herbivores, carnivores, those that eat by power of their dexterity, and the domesticated — live in both dry and wet places. These categories are important for explaining the respective potencies of their flesh.

The flesh of animals that live in dry places is cool, light, and coarse, due to which it clears away fever involved with wind and phlegm, the phlegm factor being predominant. The flesh of animals that live in wet places is oily, heavy, and warm; thus, it helps disorders of the stomach, kidneys, the lower back, cold disorders, and cold and wind disorders. The flesh of animals that live in both places has both capacities in the sense that it has the capacity to clear away heat disorders that involve phlegm and wind as well as cold-wind disorders.

The flesh of large birds, of animals that get food by the power of their dexterity, and those that eat raw flesh is rough, light, and sharp; thereby, it generates digestive fire, and because it is rough, it destroys tumors. It also increases flesh and clears away all cold disorders.

The flesh of sheep is oily and warm due to which it is easy to digest, increases physical strength, and furthers all seven physical constituents. It clears away wind and phlegm and increases appetite.

Goat meat is heavy and cool; hence, it serves to aggravate accumulations of all three humors. It is effective against a certain venereal disease [syphilis?] the source of which is trees and which is communicated through intercourse between the sexes. Goat meat also helps against smallpox[146] and sores that arise from being burned by fire.

The flesh of cows and bulls — beef — is cool and oily and clears away fevers associated with wind. The flesh from the area of the backbone of horses, the wild ass, donkey, and young mules eliminates the flowing of pus from any part of the body, inside or outside. It clears away cold disorders of the kidneys, the small of the back, and so forth as well as lymph disorders.

Pork is cool and light. It will cause sores or wounds to heal and is helpful for brown phlegm diseases [including tuberculosis].

Water buffalo is very warm, whereby it will increase sleep and flesh; it is not good. Yak flesh is oily and warm, due to which it clears away cold disorders and will generate a little blood and bile.

House birds and hopping house birds increase semen and help sores — any type of sore, wound, or abrasion. The flesh of peacocks helps with eye diseases. If your throat is blocked, it helps to unclog it. If you eat it, you will not age so easily.

Wild yak clears away cold disorders of the stomach and liver and generates digestive fire. The flesh of most larger herbivorous animals is cool and light, thus helping to clear away heat disorders that involve phlegm. Rabbit flesh is rough due to which it generates warmth and stops diarrhea.

Marmot flesh is oily and heavy, and hence warming. It will help chronic sores that are difficult to treat and helps cold-wind disorders as well as problems of the kidneys, the small of the back, and even chronic head disorders.

The flesh of the otter is an aphrodisiac; it clears away cold disorders of the kidneys and the small of the back. In general, fish clears away disorders of the stomach, increases appetite, clears sight, and helps to clear away abrasions and chronic sores. It breaks apart phlegm that has stuck together.

There are further differences among the capacities of these meats by way of whether the animal is male or female and whether the meat is from the upper or lower part of the body. Flesh from the lower part of a male animal and from the upper part of a female animal is lighter; flesh from any part of a pregnant animal is heavier. The flesh of female animals that go on four feet, such as cows, is lighter as is the flesh of all types of male birds. With regard to any animal, flesh from the head, upper part of the body [i.e., shoulders], chest, hips, lower back, and legs is respectively heavier as you go down the list.

With regard to the seven constituents, blood is heavier than the nutritional essence; flesh is heavier than blood; fat is heavier than flesh; bone is heavier than fat; marrow is heavier than bone, and the regenerative fluid is heavier than marrow. Their heaviness is in the respective order of the list of seven.

Fresh meat is cool, whereas dried meat — in Tibet it is not cooked and dried, only dried — is warm and more nutritious. One-year-old meat is particularly warm due to which it suppresses wind and generates digestive fire. Uncooked, frozen, or roasted meat is more difficult to digest, and its potency is heavy, whereas dried meat and well boiled meat is light and easier to digest.

Question: What about organ meats?
Answer: Their potencies are explained in a section on medicines made from substances taken from animals. It explains about horns, hair, brain, bone, liver, lungs, kidneys, spleen, stomach, large intestine, etc. It explains the capacities of these in terms of three topics: correspondences, relative strength of the five elements, and dependent-arisings. For instance, in terms of the capacity that arises from a correspondence, the kidneys of any animal will help in any kidney disease, and eating the brains of an animal will help someone with a brain problem. Incidentally, someone who has the particular disease called phlegm-wind dizziness should eat the brain of a sheep, and someone with epilepsy should eat the brain of a sheep with particular medicine added in it.

13 Diet: Oils, Herbs, and Cooking

Next is the topic of oils:[147] butter, grain oils, marrow, and fat. The taste of all these is sweet. Fat is heavier and cooler than marrow, marrow is heavier and cooler than oil, and oil is heavier and cooler than butter. Since oils are oily, blunt, soft, subtle, pliant, and moist, they are helpful to counteract the weakness of the old and the young and helpful for those with little physical strength of any age, the emaciated, those whose skin is rough, those whose regenerative fluid is spent, and those who have had much diarrhea and so forth. They are also helpful for wind disorders that arise from too much verbal or mental activity and so forth.

New butter is cool; it helps with virility, improves one's color and strength, and clears away bilious heat disorders. Old butter that has aged for a year has curative power for the insane, the forgetful, those who are apt to faint, and those with sores.

Clarified butter, or ghee, which is made by boiling butter that has not aged too much and removing the impurities that collect at the surface, makes your intelligence sharp, clears the faculty of memory, produces warmth greatly in the body, generates physical strength, and increases life span. Clarified butter is the supreme of oils, having thousands of capacities.

In Tibet we drink clarified butter a lot. We boil it in the evening, remove the impurities, then maybe add some honey or sugar, and drink it in place of tea — even a big cup. Take it when it is still hot, like tea. One reason why we Tibetans are oily is this: Right after a child is born, we take a stick that has the syllable *dhīḥ*, which is the seed syllable of Mañjushrī, the manifestation of the wisdom of all Buddhas, carved on it. We stick it into a yellow powdered substance that is taken from the liver of an elephant and is like musk, and put it on the child's tongue, thereby leaving the yellow letter *dhīḥ*. This is for the purpose of setting up the dependent-arising of the generation of a bright mind and clever tongue. Then, even before the mother's milk is given, approximately one teaspoonful of melted butter with a little molasses or honey is given to the child. This is why we Tibetans are so oily — why we have such shining complexions.

I did this for the child of an American that I delivered in Dharmsala, and now that child's face is oilier than the usual Westerner. We have a saying that if the face of a child is very white and not very oily, the mother must have been very poor as she could not have had the chance to give the baby this butter treatment after birth.

Question: Would a person with bile problems not be harmed by drinking butter?

Answer: In winter it would not harm, but Tibetans are so used to drinking it that it does not harm even at other times. In Tibet the tantric monks drink three to four cups a day whereas others have a single cup. A sharp mind and clear memory bring more introspection as well as the ability to keep things in mind. If even though you have a clear mind you do not have sharp memory, you cannot keep your mind on what you are thinking.

To repeat, butter increases warmth, strength, and life span, and brings about the supreme physical oiliness. It is very potent and has thousands of functions.

A cheese-like product made from the milk of a cow that has just given birth as well as cheeses made from whey and other milk products are all good for relieving loss of appetite, constipation due to dried feces, and phlegm. The "butter" that naturally gathers on the sides of a wooden milk pail clears away phlegm-wind disorders and generates digestive fire.

More particularly, beyond the powers of the "butter" just mentioned, butter from "dri" and from sheep also has the potency of clearing away cold and wind disorders. The butter of the "dzo", the cross-breed where the father is a yak and the mother is a cow, is neutral, neither hot nor cold; therefore, we consider it the best. The butter of the cow and goat is cool and, therefore, clears heat disorders that are associated with wind. These descriptions are in terms of new butter; when it has aged for a year, even cow and goat butter are warm and, therefore, clear away cold and wind disorders.

Among grain oils, oil from white and black sesame have a hot and sharp potency, producing flesh for skinny people but reducing flesh in those who are stocky. In our system there are some fantastic things, such as that one food, when eaten, produces different results depending on the person. When white or black sesame oil is eaten in food or rubbed on the body, it makes your body firm, whether you are fat or thin, and clears away wind associated with phlegm.

Question: Do you ever drink sesame oil?
Answer: We first use it in cooking, such as in deep-frying bread, and then drink it, at which time it is quite palatable; otherwise, it is not palatable. Drink it when it is drinkably hot. For somebody who has a lot of wind, it is very helpful; however, those with a lot of bile should not take it.

White or black mustard seed oil suppresses wind but generates phlegm and bile. Mustard generates a lot of bile.

If you put half a teaspoonful in your food, it normally would not harm, but four teaspoons all the time would be harmful.

Marrow in any form overcomes wind and increases the strength of the regenerative fluid, but it will increase phlegm a little. In general, fat helps with pain in the joints and bones as well as with burned skin, no matter how it is burned. Fat can also be used in an application for burns. It helps to overcome wind disorders, helps when "yellow fluid" comes out the ear, helps with brain disorders, and clears away womb disorders.

Persons who are predominantly bilious should drink clarified new butter whereas those who are predominantly phlegmic should drink clarified aged butter and those with predominant wind should drink sesame oil. People who use such oils, and especially clarified butter, frequently and steadily will cause their internal warmth to flame up and the empty places in the body to become clean — these will not fill up with lymph and so forth. Also, all seven physical constituents will be very firm, physical strength will be generated, a good color will be created, and the senses will be steady. They will not grow old so easily, being able to live for a hundred years.

Question: Why is oiliness so desirable?
Answer: First, when you eat food, the nutritional essence turns into blood, then blood into flesh, flesh to fat, fat to bone, bone to marrow, and the very fatty marrow turns into the essence of essences which has its seat at the heart but pervades the whole body. The latter has the capacity of generating physical strength, physical magnificence, good color, and strength of activity. Taking oil increases the capacity of the marrow.

Question: Is oiliness of the skin representational of how strong the marrow is?
Answer: Yes, exactly. It is a sign of good marrow. That is why I spoke earlier about putting butter into a baby's

mouth even before it takes its mother's milk.

Question: What type of butter should a phlegmic type take?
Answer: Aged but not rotten butter; "aged" means that it has stayed for a year. You could put it in the refrigerator or freezer; that would make it aged.

Question: What are seasonal uses of fats?
Answer: In the summer and winter you should make more use of grain oils. In the spring you should use aged butter and in the fall new butter.

Other types of oil from "fruits" such as walnuts and from seeds such as peach seeds are described in a separate section on fruits in the textbook.

HERBS

Within the topic of herbs and plants[148] there is a group of hot tasting ones such as garlic, onions, and so forth, and a group of bitter ones such as dandelion and a type of dandelion that grows in the woods, is tall, and has many flowers unlike common dandelion. Furthermore, herbs and plants can be divided into those that grow in dry and in wet places. They are used dry, wet, cooked with other things, or raw; within this last list, the former are warm and light, whereas the latter are cool and heavy, due to which they have the qualities of clearing away, respectively, cold disorders and heat disorders.

Onions and garlic increase sleep and appetite and clear away phlegm-wind disorders. White garlic is heavy and cool whereby it clears away diseases brought on by organisms and clears away heat disorders. Due to its coolness it clears away heat disorders and disorders of organisms; due to its heaviness it clears away wind disorders.

A young white radish — "young" means still small, before the 15th of July — is light and warm; it generates digestive fire and clears away all three humors. However, a mature white radish that has been stored in a cool place is heavy and cool and generates phlegm and so forth. Turnip is similar but is helpful in protecting against all sicknesses that come from poisons.

All types of mountain garlic are difficult to digest, increase appetite, and are heavy. Himalayan rhubarb ("jum")[149] and "chulo" [sorrel leaves],[150] grow in mountains; the first one has a stalk, the second one does not. The first grows like bamboo such that when it gets old the stalk is hollow; the second does not have a long stalk and has big leaves on top, which get reddish as it gets older. The taste of "chulo" is sour and astringent; "jum" is both sweet and sour. They both clear away phlegm and increase appetite.

All these herbs and plants block up the passageways of the channels and make medicine less potent; this is why we tell people taking medicine not to eat herbs. When you eat them, the openings of the channels constrict.

COOKING

Concerning mixing and cooking foods, rice soup is of three varieties — thinner, less thin, and thick; there is also just cooked rice, not in the form of soup.[151] The former among these are lighter and easier to digest; they get heavier as you go down the list — the thin soup is lighter, the thicker one is heavier.

The thinner variety clears away thirst and causes the humors to come into balance; it dispells emaciation, equalizes the physical constituents, generates heat, and makes the insides of the channels flexible. The more viscous rice group generates warmth, can clear both hunger and thirst, and gradually restores a weakened body. Also, it will clear away the leftovers of illnesses as well as constipation due to blockage of gas. The most viscous rice soup will stop diarrhea, generate appetite, and clear away thirst. Therefore, rice soup is praised highly for those who have had dysentery, to restore their strength and to get rid of the illness. In all of its forms, rice soup is praised. Other gruels are similar.

Rice boiled in meat broth or in milk becomes heavy. Boiled in water, it is light and easy to digest. Popped rice — the rice is washed, dried a little, put in a little bit of oil, and popped such that it is very crunchy — stops diarrhea and helps to mend broken bones.

Soup made from immature grains will constipate and will overcome digestive fire; therefore, it is very bad. People like to take corn and roast it incompletely or break open a pea pod and eat it when it is not completely mature. Such is not good for you.

Parched grains — which have been put in a pan and parched — in soup are really good; they are light, soft, warm, easy to digest, and very palatable. In Tibet we put barley in a pan with sand in it, heat it, and then separate the grain from the sand. Thus, it is cooked nicely; then, it is used in soup; it is excellent. To parch it, we wash the barley in water, dry it in the sun to keep it moist on the inside, then parch it in the hot sand whereupon it is separated from the sand and put into a big container. People then step on it, separating off the husk; then, it is thrown in the wind to clean it.

Ground parched barley, when eaten cold, generates physical strength and is heavy. Even though it is heavy, when eaten cold, it is light and soft when cooked, due to which it is easy to digest.

Leftovers after many days will overpower the digestive fires of the stomach. In general, it is said that after twenty-four hours any food is stale.[152] Even in a refrigerator, the cold causes it to come into this class. "Stale food" means that it has the capacity of cold. Also, when you freeze foods, their entities will not remain the same; some will become warmer, some colder. If you freeze foods raw, they will remain the same, but if you cook and then freeze them, they have already changed. The potency of raw, frozen meat will get warmer in nature if you leave it in the freezer for several months, but it will not rot or hurt you.

Question: Does the same thing apply to foods that are cooked and then canned or preserved?
Answer: There is no way that the capacity of food can remain the same in a can. There is also the factor of the "rust" of the metal of the can. The "rust" of the metal can help with diseases of the liver and eyes; thus, there sometimes can be some help too.

Question: Is it a good idea to cook rice and keep it in the refrigerator for a few days?
Answer: It is not good; if you cook it twice, it gets heavier and colder. If you cook enough for three days and take it out as you need it, it gets heavier and more difficult to digest.

Question: What about bread?
Answer: There is nothing wrong with cooking bread and eating it after a few days; the degeneration of food of which I am speaking is in terms of food cooked with water, whereas bread is baked.

Question: Western nutritionists say that rice by itself does not supply a proper diet.
Answer: Usually, we eat something else with rice — meat and so forth — but rice soup is good for someone who has just had dysentery. Even in rice soup you would put vegetables.

Question: Is garlic used to treat heart disease?
Answer: If the heart problem is a wind disorder or a phlegm-wind disorder with an involvement of organisms and not a blood disorder, then garlic will help. However, if it is a wind and blood disorder — a heat disorder — it will not help.

Question: How would refrigeration affect vegetables?
Answer: It is about the same for vegetables as for grains.

Even if you heat them after taking them out of the refrigerator, they have already become heavier because of being made cold. Meat, however, will get warmer in potency. Getting warmer means that it is getting heavier. Fresh meat is cool and light; old meat is warm and heavy.

Ground, parched barley mixed with hot water, tea, or beer and thereby made into a soup is easy to digest and will make you thinner; it clears away all faults of the three humors.

Ground, parched barley can be made into a more pasty mixture like dough and made to ferment, yielding barley beer. This clears away wind problems and helps with internal heat, digestive fire. If this beer has aged, it will increase appetite and clear away all problems of the humors. However, sour items can harm the heart a little if you take too much, since they increase blood.

All types of meat broth will restore a degenerated body, will cause physical satisfaction, and will help with wind problems.

Then, there is a product from ground parched barley made into dough and left for a day; it becomes a little sour. Make it into flat pieces like noodles; put them out to dry, and then put them into soup. This is praised as supreme for counteracting wind.

Greens
Nettle leaves will overcome wind and generate warmth. However, if you eat a lot, they will rise up phlegm and bile problems.

The leaves of mallow,[153] a plant with a big red flower, are very helpful for stopping diarrhea; they will generate heat. An herb called *Plantago major*[154] that, when cut, is bloodlike inside performs the same functions.

There is a white tuber, like a potato, which has a long stalk with a yellow flower at the top;[155] it is given to pigs for food. Its leaves overcome wind problems and cause abrasions to dry, but they generate phlegm and bile.

The leaves of a plant called "nayu",[156] which have the potency of mercury, harm the eyes, but they open up the intestinal passage when one is constipated due to blockage of wind.

There is a red-leaved plant about two feet high,[157] which we commonly call the "new year flower".[158] Its leaves clear away problems of all three humors. It is used as a food dye — very bright red.

Something like a dandelion called "gyap"[159] which grows in the woods and has three flowers to a stalk and dandelion[160] itself — i.e., the leaves — are cool and therefore clear away heat problems. The reference is to new dandelion leaves, when the plant is young.

The leaves of ginger[161] which has a round type of leaf and grows in snow mountains or in stony areas on mountains where there used to be snow clear away bilious heat disorders and head problems brought on by bile.

The leaves of all types of beans or peas increase appetite but generate problems of phlegm and wind. They will cause oil to come out of the body and will clear away undigested grain oils, such as sesame. The leaves of peas and beans, when new, are neutral in terms of heat and cold and will in time generate wind-phlegm problems and small sores on the body.

Eating mustard leaves will disturb phlegm and bile. A leaf called "ja-wa",[162] Angelica root, that grows where dandelions are and a larger leaf called "ra-nay"[163] that grows in the woods will clear away phlegm-wind.

The leaves of a big white radish[164] are hot in potency; they generate heat, stop diarrhea, and help wind. After the autumnal equinox they lose this capacity due to becoming too mature. White garlic and blue garlic[165] as well as their leaves are helpful for wind disorders.

Salt, Pepper, And So Forth
Salt brings out the taste of all foods, generates digestive heat, is easy to digest, makes it easy to defecate, and so

forth. There are many types of salt; I do not think the salt you use here has these capacities whereas pure sea salt would.

Guinea pepper[166] opens up the doors of the channels and generates phlegm and wind. It is hot and causes your tongue to become tingly, not the way red pepper does. Ginger[167] generates digestive heat. Asafoetida[168] overcomes wind disorders. All spices bring out the taste of foods and increase appetite.

DRINK

Drink has many subsections — milk, water, beer, etc.[169] Milk clears away wind; water clears away bile, and beer clears away phlegm. In opposite order, milk generates phlegm; water generates wind, and beer generates bile.

The taste of most milks is sweet; their post-digestive taste is also sweet. Milks are oily and heavy, due to which they increase the seven physical constituents, generate magnificent tone, clear away wind and bile problems, increase virility, and generate phlegm. Therefore, ultimately at the end of digestion, milk makes one more virile and at that point is cool and heavy.

Cow milk mainly helps the lungs. It helps with chronic cold disorders, among which diabetes is included, and is a supreme of essence-extracts for increasing sharpness of mind, a mother's milk, the physical constituents, and so forth. Goat milk mainly clears away uncomfortable breathing as in asthma, hayfever, etc. Sheep milk overcomes wind problems but can harm the heart in that it can cause palpitations, since it increases blood if taken in excessive quantities.

"Dri" milk worsens diseases of phlegm and bile. Nevertheless, in a cool, high land such as Tibet it is not harmful; we consider "dri" milk to be superior. Horse and donkey milk restore the lungs but will make your mind a little dull.

Fresh cold milk, that is to say, fresh milk that has not been heated, is heavy and cool and will increase organisms and phlegm. If you just bring it to a boil, it becomes lighter and warmer. However, if you boil it down, it becomes heavy and difficult to digest. If you take milk right from the cow while still warm, it is like ambrosia — very suitable for the body.

If you have an imbalance of heat or cold or have frequent common colds, skim milk — which is left over after the butter has been taken out — will make it go one way or the other. Also, it will cause a moving sickness to locate in its own place. Then, you can take medicine to get rid of the disease.

The taste and post-digestive taste of all yogurts are sour. Yogurt is cool and oily; it helps if you are constipated. It will clear away wind fevers and generates appetite.

* * *

Following is a list of foods randomly put to Dr. Donden for brief identifications:

FOOD	TASTE	POTENCY
FRUITS		
Banana	sweet	heavy and oily
Orange	sour and sweet	cool and light
Grapefruit	sweet	very heavy
Grapes	sweet	very heavy
Apple	sweet	heavy and cool
Strawberry	sour	coarse and cool
Peach	sweet	very heavy
Tomato	sour and sweet	light and sour
Watermelon	sweet	cool and very heavy
Coconut	sweet	oily and heavy
Pineapple	sweet and sour	coarse and heavy
Raisin	sweet	cool and slightly lighter than pineapple
Lemon	sour	cool and coarse

VEGETABLES

Carrots	sweet	heavy
Celery	bitter	light
Lettuce	semi-sweet	heavy
Spinach	bitter	light and hot
Green Pepper	hot	sharp and coarse
Hot Pepper	hot	sharp and coarse
Eggplant	semi-sweet	hot and heavy
Red Cabbage	sweet	heavy
Peas	sweet	heavy
Mushrooms	astringent & sweet	hot and heavy
Potato	sweet	heavy
Sweet Potato	sweet	heavy
Corn	sweet	heavy
Onion	sweet and salty	hot and heavy

GRAINS

White rice	sweet	light and cool
Brown rice	sweet	slightly heavier
Rye	sweet	heavy and cool
Wheat	sweet	heavy and cool
Wheat bread	sweet	heavy and cool

NUTS/SEEDS

Peanuts	sweet	oily, hot & heavy
Walnuts	sweet	oily, hot & heavy
Sesame seeds	sweet	oily, hot & heavy
Sesame butter	sweet	oily, hot & heavy
Peanut butter	sweet	oily, hot & heavy

DAIRY PRODUCTS

Yogurt	sour	coarse
Cheese	sour	coarse
Cow's milk	sweet	cool and light
Butter	sweet	oily, hot, and heavy

Ice cream	sweet	cool and heavy

MEAT

Salty fish (anchovies)	sweet	heavy and hot
Pork	sweet	cool and light
Mutton	sweet	heavy and warm
Beef	sweet	cool and light
Chicken	sweet	very light
Fish	sweet	heavy and hot

CONDIMENTS

Black Pepper	hot	hot and coarse
Salt	salty	heavy
Sugar	sweet	very cool and light
Honey	sweet	light and dry
Garlic	sweet	hot and heavy
Soy Sauce	salty	oily

MISCELLANEOUS

Alcohol	sweet and bitter	very hot and light
Dark and light beer	sweet and bitter	cool and light
Tofu (soy bean curd)	sweet	heavy and oily
Eggs	sweet	heavy and hot

1. Foods with sweet taste are good for wind and harmful for phlegm.
2. Sour-sweet taste: good for wind and blood.
3. Sour taste: good for phlegm and harmful for wind.
4. Salty taste: good for phlegm and wind; harmful for bile and blood.
5. Bitter taste: good for bile and harmful for wind.
6. Astringent taste: good for phlegm.

14 Questions

Question: Do you have medicine for allergies?

Answer: Many foreigners have come to me in India to be treated for certain allergies, and the treatment has been successful. The signs of this disease are sneezing and itching; in the worst form, it stops your voice. There are five varieties according to the predominance of wind, phlegm, bile, blood, and a mixture of phlegm and wind. You should not eat raw scallions but should eat honey. There are powdered medicines, pills, and decoctions for· treatment.

Question: Are there any complications with using contraception and birth control devices?

Answer: In our medicine system, we have contraceptive means that last for a whole lifetime and others that are temporary, but we do not allow use of these except for people who have had seven or eight children. Contraception is not so bad from the point of view of religion, because you are not killing anyone. Even though contraception stops someone from coming into the womb, you would not be throwing anyone out who had already gotten into the womb and so you do not have the fault of murder. Still, you would have the lesser fault of not allowing the consciousness to enter the womb. If you take medicine in order to expel a child that has formed in the womb, that has the greater fault of committing murder.

Question: What about organ transplants?
Answer: For the eyes this is very good. However, I doubt what is being done with kidneys because I think that our medicines for restoring kidneys are very successful. I do not think kidney transplants will be very helpful since it is not your own kidney.

Still, the donor of an organ will receive the virtue of having given it to someone else. If the person gives the gift of an eye or a portion of the eye with the wish that all sentient beings could attain the eye of wisdom and so forth, that person will achieve great merit with great fruits. When you give with such special good thoughts, it is all the more powerful. Just giving it without such special thought would lead to your having great resources in a future life as, say, a human, but when it is dedicated to highest enlightenment, it can bear tremendous fruit.

Question: Is giving blood regularly, every month or every two months, harmful to the body?
Answer: In a general way, if you give blood even without any of these special thoughts, you will have a good body in future lives. If you give it with special thoughts of altruistic dedication to highest enlightenent, then it is even better.

If your body is in good shape and your blood is in good shape, you could give blood every month. It depends on your condition as well as the circumstances of those who need the blood. Medically speaking, you should give blood within the context of not doing it to the point where it harms your own body.

Question: What do you recommend about fasting?
Answer: Fasting is good for a person who is in good physical

condition and has excessive phlegm and oil. In general, fasting should be at a time when one has too much phlegm, too much oil, and is not digesting well. If, during the fast, you take water with a little lemon juice, this helps in getting rid of phlegm.

Question: What foods should one eat when coming off a fast?

Answer: When you leave a fast, you should eat light food, something that is easy to digest, such as rice soup. In the Tibetan way of fasting, for a month from the fifth day of the third month to the sixteenth of the fourth month, there might be two or three hundred people fasting. Before sunrise you get up, wash, and perform the religious recitations that you normally do. Then, we do recitations together on this first day and recite mantra; except for reciting mantra, we give up talking. On that day, not only do you not eat any food but also you do not drink any fluid at all. Also, you would not spit. You spend the day reciting texts, reciting mantra, and meditating. Then, at night you go to sleep, and the next morning you take some sour yogurt or lemon juice with a little water. Then, you do your recitations, drinking Tibetan tea with salt, milk, and butter in it. At sunrise, you could take some noodle soup, also drinking tea during the day. At noon you eat enough food to fill the stomach. Then, until you go to bed that evening you do not eat.

The next morning you just take tea with salt, milk, and butter in it; you do not speak except to recite; you also do many prostrations to the Buddha, Doctrine, and Spiritual Community. Then, the following morning you not only drink tea upon rising but also, at sunrise, take noodle soup with meat in it. Thus, you have noodle soup every other day for the rest of the month. In the morning on the days that you eat, you take noodle soup and at noon eat some food, for instance, ground parched barley that is mixed with fluid to make it into a paste and then fried. Melted butter is put on it, and molasses; these are for the sake of not generating wind, for when you fast, you tend to get more wind.

In accordance with your physical condition, it is possible to go with a mixture of water and lemon juice for maybe even three days, but more likely two days, or one day. But to go for ten days this way is a completely different situation concerned with special religious practices; I am talking about fasting for physical purposes.

The best time to fast is in the spring or just at the period between fall and winter. Not everyone should fast; those persons predominated by wind should not fast. Those who can use fasting are phlegmic by nature having an excess of oil.

Question: Why are the two times, spring and between fall and winter, good for fasting?
Answer: In the winter, because it is cold, your pores tend to be closed and the phlegmic substances are held in the body. Then in spring these begin to melt, and thus spring is a good time to fast to get rid of these.

The period between fall and winter is when fruits and vegetables and so forth have ripened and their capacity is returning back to the ground. Similarly, internally you fast in order to cause the oily elements to dry. Inside and outside thereby come into accord.

Question: Would fasting help hay fever?
Answer: As mentioned earlier, there are five varieties of hay fever; for the phlegmic type, fasting could help. Otherwise not.

Question: Americans are very weight-conscious, and people are always dieting to lose weight. What is your opinion about this?
Answer: It is not good to be very fat. According to our medical texts, exercise is not very helpful as a means to lose weight even though it is basically salutary; rather, we emphasize taking care of diet.

Question: Is this a case of reducing the amount you eat?
Answer: No. You should not reduce the amount you eat. I can explain this from my own experience. In the West and in India there are many fat people who seek to reduce by not eating any meat, just eating one or two things, maybe just eating potato or just a few foods. This is completely wrong, a great mistake. For, if you eat food that is not nutritious, it will increase the lymph and phlegm in your body, and you will get fatter and weaker. The reason why there are not too many fat Tibetans, I think, is that our diet is better. We eat nutritious food and engage in vigorous physical activity.

If you want to be thin, you should drink fluid before eating and then, after eating, not drink much fluid. If you want to remain as you are, you should take fluid along with the meal. If you want to be fatter, you should eat first and take fluid afterward; for instance, after the meal take a cup of beer with honey in it. If you want to lose weight, before the meal take a cup of boiled hot water with honey in it; boil the water, cool it off, and then add in a little honey.

Question: Do you think that joggers are wasting their time?
Answer: Jogging can be helpful for the body if proper diet is enacted simultaneously because it makes your body more healthy, firm, strong. Still, the main thing is food; for instance, you cannot operate a car without gas. If you do not eat well and go out and exercise, it will ruin your body, but if you eat well and exercise well, you will be in good health and strong.

If you are of windy nature and go on an empty stomach, this increases wind and will probably lead to mental problems as well as other physical diseases. The nature of wind is light and moving; it is also rough; when you fast, these qualities are increased.

Question: What about taking wine with meals?
Answer: Alcohol in general is harmful to the liver; so, aside

from taking a little bit in the winter, it is not a good substance to be taking. The liver is one of the main organs of the body.

Question: Why was surgery stopped?
Answer: At the time of King Tri-song-de-dzen in the eighth century, an operation was performed on the mother of Mu-tri-dzen-bo. She died from the operation. The king prohibited the practice of surgery in Tibet, and at that time, whatever the king said had to be done. That is one reason.

The other reason is that from the religious point of view and from many other points of view, surgery is not that good. From the religious point of view, it is preferable to undergo the illness and take medicine to cure it than it would be to seek to avoid the illness and be operated upon. If the disease is caused by one of your own earlier actions, you should undergo the result. Otherwise, you might have to go through it by being reborn as a hell-being, for instance, and it will be all the worse. From the point of view of temporary physical health also, it is better to cure the organ than to remove it.

Question: Is it not the same to take medicine or have surgery? In both cases you are getting rid of the illness that is to be experienced.
Answer: There is a difference. It may look on the surface as if taking medicine is similar to surgery, but when you take medicine, you are doing it in a soft or peaceful way whereas with surgery you are just removing it.

Doctors or special priests also perform meditative rituals in which the pills are dissolved into the emptiness of inherent existence and then reappear as deities who dissolve into ambrosia. Because the pills have been blessed this way into a magnificent state, anyone who is still breathing can benefit from them. Most Tibetans, as they are about to die, know they are going to die; so, they take special blessed pills. A pill is dissolved in water, and the person takes a little just before dying.

Question: Are accessory therapies such as moxa widely used nowadays?
Answer: Accessory therapies must be used because their purpose is to keep the disease from coming back. There are two kinds of accessory therapy in general: soft and rough. The rougher are moxabustion, acupuncture, letting blood, and also the letting of lymph from the joints. Among the softer are applications of ointments, massage, putting on hot compresses (medicines in cloth), going to a hot spring or if you are in a place where there is no hot spring, you can do the equivalent with medicine — the medicines are boiled and then put in a big tub; the person then enters the tub.

Question: Do Tibetan doctors also take care of bones?
Answer: Just one doctor does everything. For instance, in India a person came to me who had broken his thigh bone falling down stairs. The Indian doctors said they would have to cut off the leg. I treated him, and the fellow is going about nowadays; he has healed. There are splints and also mending medicines.

Also, an elderly woman fell down a set of steep stairs in Dharmsala and broke her collarbone. They brought her to the Indian hospital where they said all that they could do was to lessen her pain. The next day they brought her to me. I put on the Tibetan type of plaster and wood splint and gave her medicine; after four or five months she was restored. Thus, I can say from my own experience that we do not need a separate doctor for treating bones.

There is medicine taken orally for the sake of reducing pain, reducing inflammation, and stopping sores from developing, and then medicine that causes quick knitting of the bone in that region as well as the channels [nerves]. From the outside, first we set the bone carefully. Then, medicine is put on from the outside, and a splint is wrapped with cloth and plaster. You can cause the mending of a bone that is broken more easily than one that is cracked.

Question: What about teeth?
Answer: For teeth we analyze to see whether the cause is sinusitis or organisms. We then give medicine to kill the organisms or to treat the sinusitis.

Question: Is it possible to study Tibetan medicine without studying Buddhism? Can you separate the two?
Answer: It is definitely best to do both together. The medical system is intimately involved with Buddhism. It is a Buddhist science, part of the Secret Mantra teaching. Understanding one branch of the teaching helps in understanding the others.

Question: What about fast food?
Answer: If the meat that you get in a hamburger is meat, if the bread is bread, if the vegetable is vegetable, and if the milk in a milkshake is milk, you are at least getting those. However, for someone like myself who is not used to such food, it does not suffice. I think there is a factor of being accustomed to it. It is said that you can get used to things such that they will not harm you. Since I am not accustomed to such food, I either throw up or have diarrhea. A peacock can even eat poison as food.

Question: Is it possible that Americans are becoming adapted to eating preservatives and food additives and they will no longer be harmful to us?
Answer: When food has additives or when potent fertilizers are used, I do not find such foods to have their usual taste or potency, but I think you are used to them. In Tibet, there was one type of meat to which we added spices to keep it from rotting; otherwise, we did not use additives because they take away the natural potency of the food.

Question: What do you think about chemotherapy for the

treatment of cancer?
Answer: I have the suspicion that although chemotherapy could temporarily destroy a tumor, it will generate another problem.

Question: From your visit to America, what do you think is the most unhealthy element in American life?
Answer: I think that although your food in general is very good, you tend to put sugar in everything. It is almost as if you use sugar as most people use salt; you even put it in hot pepper sauces. You have gotten used to so much sugar that you just keep eating more and more and more of it. It will induce cold diseases, such as diabetes, as well as rheumatism; it will also make great problems in old age. It increases the potency of various organisms in the body that bring out tumors and so forth. For instance, I will be talking to you about seven types of organisms, the first type being invisible, the second type being visible to a microscope, and the rest visible to the eye. Sweet things increase the potency of these organisms.

SELECTED TOPICS

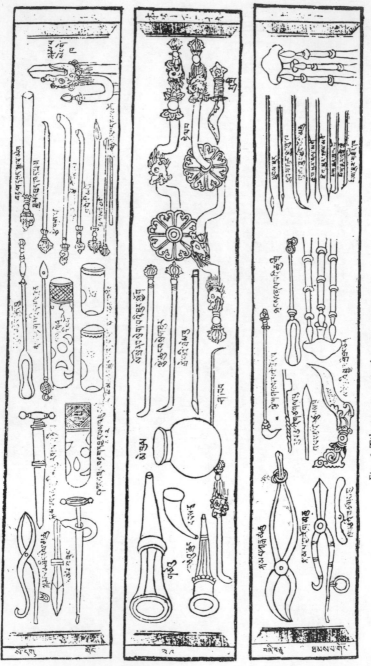

Fig. 6 Tibetan surgical instruments.

15 Diabetes

Diabetes is included among chronic degenerative urinary disorders involving frequent urination.[170] The initial signs or precursors of the disease are that after sleeping, one's bed clothes are damp particularly near the genitals, one perspires a great deal — the perspiration having a bad odor — hair and nails grow quickly, mouth and throat are dry, one is frequently thirsty and likes to eat and drink cool things, the palms of the hands and the soles of the feet have a hot burning sensation which, nevertheless, is not painful, when urinating the last part is more dense, and the urine attracts more flies than usual. In the early stages of the disease the character of the urine is indefinite; therefore, not much can be told from the urine.

With regard to the actual signs of such a chronic degenerative urinary disorder, when it arises from phlegm problems, food is not digested well, appetite is stopped, one sleeps a lot, one's body feels heavy, there is much mucus in the mouth, and one is nauseous. When it arises from bile problems, one's genitals and urinary bladder burn during urination and one has a dry mouth, a sense of great heat in the body, diarrhea, and susceptibility to the common cold. When it arises from wind problems, the heart palpitates, one is unable to sleep much, has difficulty in breathing, an unreasonable sense of fright from time to time, and a great deal of mucus in the mouth, and is ravenous.

In general, the urine of a patient with this disease has a sediment that can be of several different varieties: like milk when it is due to phlegm problems, like molasses or sugarcane soup, like rice soup, smelly and sticky like bean thread and cold to the touch, and like the saliva of a cow or elephant — the drool of a cow or elephant. The urine can be black, blue, yellow, red, or orange. Its taste is sweet like honey; with treatment, however, the urine loses its sweet taste. In cases of bile and blood problems, the urine has an unpleasant odor.

With respect to the main causes of the disease, in terms of diet it is brought on by too much food that is salty, sweet, having cool potency, and having a heavy nature. In terms of behavior, it is brought on by staying a long time in damp places. Due to these conditions, phlegm and fat increase.

In terms of treatment, there is medicine for the disease in general as well as for the particular phlegm, bile, or wind problem in particular. If the disease goes untreated, various sores, bumps, and tumors will appear.

Question: Are such patients fat?
Answer: Most Indians who have this disease are fat; among Tibetans, however, it varies. Tibetans are less susceptible than Indians because even though Tibetans put a little salt in tea and in food, they do not eat many sweets. Indians, however, in general eat many sweets, particularly sugar.

Question: What is the nature of the medicines?
Answer: They contain mainly tree bark, flowers, and fruits. The only animal product is musk. The ingredients for the medicines are nowadays gathered mainly from the Himalayas, near Tibet.

Question: Between aged and young patients, which are more

likely to die of this disease?
Answer: There is no definiteness with regard to which age group will die more frequently.

Question: What behavior and foods should be avoided when one has this disease?
Answer: One should not stay in cold and damp places. The worst foods are sugar, carrots, cauliflower, cabbage, molasses, turnips, and sugar beets. Once cured, it is all right to take a little bit of these foods.

Question: Is blindness associated with this disease?
Answer: Blindness is not linked to this disease.

Question: Are hereditary factors involved?
Answer: Tibetan doctors do not consider this disease to be within families. We do consider leprosy to be within families.

Question: How much medicine is taken?
Answer: At first, medicine is taken three times a day — morning, noon, and evening. Later, it is only taken in the morning and evening.

Question: Are there bad reactions to the medicines?
Answer: The effectiveness of the medicine also depends on whether the doctor has made a proper diagnosis. Often doctors will adjust the content of the medicines they prescribe for patients through periodic check-ups.

Question: What is done during the initial examination of a patient?
Answer: The doctor checks the pulses, urine, eyes, tongue, and the rest of the body. Then the doctor explains the diagnosis to the patient and compares those observations with the experience of the patient.

Question: What is examined in urinalysis?
Answer: The doctor considers odor, color, bubbles, taste, qualities when fresh and warm, qualities when cooled off, and the albumin or cloud-like substance that forms in it as well as the oily substance that forms on the top. When the urine is one day old, there are three types of analysis that can be done. In Tibet, in cases when patients cannot get to the doctor, they send their urine along with a letter that describes the symptoms. From that, the doctor can prescribe medicine. Stool analysis is done infrequently. However, from the urine, a doctor can diagnose three categories of stool.

Question: What are the characteristics of pulse?
Answer: This is a very complicated topic. The doctor must know the usual or constitutional pulse of the individual, as well as differences in pulse due to season, the pulses arising from heat and cold disorders, and individual pulses associated with specific diseases.

Question: How often must a doctor see a patient?
Answer: With diseases for which the prescribed medicine is particularly dangerous, the physician must check the patient in the evening after seeing the patient in the morning. In other cases, an interval of weeks, or even a month, may be permissible.

Question: Do regenerative problems occur in this disease?
Answer: Regenerative problems are possible when a person has had such a chronic degenerative urinary disorder for a long time. A patient with blood and bile varieties of this disease may become impotent. No such problems arise in the case of the wind and phlegm varieties.

Question: Would you elaborate on what happens if the disease is not treated?
Answer: If it is not treated well when new, little bumps will

appear over the body both internally and externally. Small sores that open when scratched develop, and also sores can develop in the kidneys, urinary bladder, stomach, and so forth. The sores or swellings are sometimes high on the outside and low in the middle, sometimes high in the middle, and sometimes have small bumps on them. Those persons who develop sores inside will become stooped. The person's limbs will become hard, and the veins will become varicose. It is hard for the pus in the bumps and sores to ripen.

16 Tumors

There are two ways of discussing the topic of tumors —
under the heading of chronic tumorous disorders and under
the heading of eighteen malignant disorders that were
prophesied for the future.

Under the heading of chronic tumorous disorders, there
are six sections which I shall identify briefly. The first deals
with the causes and conditions of these disorders which are:
undigested food, organisms, increase of lymph, and staying
in a cold place. There is no way you can get a tumor *just* in
dependence on the wind humor.

With regard to diagnosis of a patient who has any of these
chronic disorders, there are sections on how to examine the
pulse and how to perform urinalysis. The pulse can be very
quick, or, in another case, it can be like the dragging of a
crippled leg. Also, as explained before, if the top of the
urine has cracks in it, this is a sign that the patient has a
tumor.

Wherever the tumor is on the body, when it first forms,
that area will be black, and when you wash it, you will find
that things stick there and that dirt quickly gathers in this
place even after washing. For all types of tumors, patients
have a sense of cold shivers. The bowels will be irregular —

for a few days having diarrhea and for a few days being constipated. Even if patients do not know they are ill, they will become thinner and weaker.

With respect to the various types of tumors, there is one type in the stomach, the source of which is undigested nutriment. There is another type in the liver that is a blood tumor. As signs of a blood tumor having formed in the liver or gall bladder, the urine will be yellow or orange, and the eyes and skin, yellow. Also, the pulse will be quick, and the body will become very warm. There will be pains in the front and back on the right side. When the tumor has formed, the flesh will turn blackish, but the eyes will remain yellow.

With regard to a tumor in the spleen, the color of the flesh in general will not change, but on the left side right above the spleen a blackish area will develop. The patient will find it difficult to digest food and will burp up a bitter fluid.

With regard to a tumor in the stomach or large intestine, that is of a phlegmic variety but is a mixture of phlegm, blood, and lymph, if it is palpated in the morning, it will pulse. If there is a tumor in the small intestine, the signs will be similar to those of a tumor in the gall bladder, but the color of the urine is brighter. The patient will also be very thirsty.

There is a type of wind tumor in the large intestine, which, because it has the nature of wind, is sometimes greater in size and sometimes smaller. There would be no way to remove it surgically because it is of the nature of wind.

In the case of a woman's developing a blood tumor due to not menstruating, she will have pains in all joints and in the womb. In cold weather the pain will be greater, and in warm weather she will not suffer as much. At times other than the point of menstruation such as in the middle of the month, there will be a blackish discharge.

The source of stone tumors in the urinary bladder is the

kidneys. With such stones, the person suffers from urinary blockage such that urination is painful.

In the lungs there are small channels where small vessel tumors can form. Thereupon, it is difficult to cough, and the patient's voice becomes noisy. The color of the flesh turns bluish or blackish; the patient becomes thin, and tends to vomit after eating.

Stones form in the kidneys due to the lack of quick movement of water through them. It is hard at first to know that the problem is there because the person does not experience any pain. One sign is that the person will find it difficult to bend.

In general, it can be said that wherever there is a tumor in the body, the surface of the body above that spot changes in color and tends to get dirty quickly.

From another point of view, tumors can form on the inside, middle, and outside of the body. In brief, tumors on the outside can occur anywhere on the outside of the skin, also on the outside of the small intestine, the stomach, the liver, spleen, kidneys, and large intestine. Internal tumors can form on the inside of the stomach, gall bladder, small intestine, and lungs. With regard to the middle, tumors can form in the liver, spleen, kidneys, and urinary bladder. It is easiest to cure external tumors, then tumors in the center; internal ones are the most difficult to cure. Those in the middle can be cured more easily relative to the internal.

This has been a brief explanation of the six sections on chronic tumorous disorders that have existed from the past.

EIGHTEEN MALIGNANT DISORDERS

Buddha also set forth eighteen types of disorders that would develop in the future due to sentient beings' engaging more in the non-virtues and due to the construction of new materials. These mainly come from the manufacture of new creations and combinations of substances. For instance, nowadays there are a great many new things to eat; also, fertilizers now are being used to cause vegetables to grow larger and more quickly. There are also many different kinds of tobaccos for people to smoke that were not present in the past. Thus, these eighteen malignant disorders have arisen mainly in dependence on these new combinations of substances.

Also, from the Buddhist point of view, this era is a time when the heads of countries and organizations are not being honest, and the people under them are also not being honest; people are deceiving each other a great deal. The clergy are becoming more like non-clergy, mixing in worldly ways and not performing their proper practices. Also, due to deprecation of religious practice, special types of beings who are protectors of religious systems are offended. Through these karmic causes, chronic troubles are engendered. Hence, the causes of these diseases derive from the three basic mental afflictions of desire, hatred, and ignorance.

Although mainly the causes are indeed the three mental afflictions just mentioned and the three humors — wind, phlegm and bile — the primary contributing conditions are to be found in seven types of organisms living in our bodies. The first is a blood organism that has no legs; it is extremely difficult to see — I think that it would be difficult to see even with a microscope. It is with the blood and thereby moves to all the important points of the channels. This is one condition for the arising of all these types of extremely degenerative, malignant disorders; it also acts as a cause for leprosy.

Then there are organisms, larger than those, that perhaps could be seen with a microscope. They are again red ones, called "red like copper".[171] In an instant it can move throughout the whole body; it can affect the entire bloodstream very quickly. The other five types of organisms can be seen with the eye.

Question: How is the existence of these organisms known?
Answer: If you mean, how do we know that they exist in

general, in the Buddhist doctrine there are many types of subtle organisms and so forth that I think are still beyond the ken of scientists. However, if you mean, how does a doctor diagnose their presence, from the second type of organism on up I think that they can be seen; the first cannot be. It is in dependence on the word of Buddha that we know of their existence.

The eating of sweet things as well as foods that are mixtures of many different tastes and potencies increases the potency of these organisms; engaging in unacceptable behavior patterns also promotes them. Wherever such a disturbance of these organisms occurs in the seven physical constituents, that constituent will diminish in force, whereby the power of these organisms increases. Due to such a causal situation, these particularly malignant diseases arise.

These diseases in their respective forms occur in the brain, small intestine, skin, joints, flesh of forearms and the calves, anywhere in the flesh, and connective tissue; the last is difficult for a physician to diagnose. When persons first get this last illness in the connective tissue, they faint and then die within seven days, with the mouth as if laughing because the connective tissue stiffens. This happens to very few people; it is one of the worst types of malignant disorders.

When the malignant disease forms in the bones in the soles of the feet and palms of the hands, it eats away, or consumes, the bones. An early symptom of its onset is that the person senselessly starts crying, becomes rough in behavior, and as if without cause vomits or has diarrhea. The outside of the body where it forms will become dirty.

The basic entities of these diseases are heat disorders. A sign of their onset is that there will be pains on the two sides of the face; the eyes will turn red; the patient's flesh will become very hot. It will seem sometimes as if there is a pain at the top of the backbone and sometimes as if there is not.

With respect to tumors in the area of the throat and mouth, they can come at the root of the tongue, the lips, inside the lips, on the palate, in the cheeks, in the area under the ears, and in the mid-throat itself. When a tumor develops in the middle of the throat, it prevents speech and obstructs eating and drinking.

There is one type of tumor in the throat called "male"; it is bulbous and flat. Another type of throat tumor is called "female"; it is convex, like a cup turned upside down. These are not throat tumors for male and female but types of tumors that are given these names. The type called "child" is many sore-like tumors, some flat and pointed like a sword, some like a half moon, and some with a lot of bumps all over like the bumps on a toad. These can be seen externally by the eye. The pulse is hot and fluttering, and the top of the urine has cracks in it. All tumors in the throat-mouth region have these qualities. Please keep in mind that I am giving just a brief summary of the text.

There is another type of tumorous swelling that can appear anywhere in the body; it has sharp pains associated with it. Wherever this disease forms, if it is a matter of predominance of blood, there will be swelling on that side; the pain will also appear on that side. Those of worst pain appear on the left side of the body.

If this type of painful tumor is associated with a wind problem, the strength of the swelling and the pain will be indefinite as will be the place where these occur. If it forms in the heart, it is very difficult to cure. It is less difficult to cure in the liver, and even less difficult to cure if it occurs in the lungs. In the spleen it is easier again, and easier if it is in the kidneys. The tumor easiest to cure occurs in the breasts and the lymph glands, under the arms.

If this problem is associated with a blood and bile disorder, then whether you eat or not you will have a sense of bitterness in the mouth, your skin will turn yellow, and sweat will come from the roots of the hair on the head. In the wind variety, the mouth is dry, the mind becomes confused, and one will yawn a lot.

As mentioned above, with regard to these painful

tumors, those that are the most difficult to cure are in the heart, liver, and lungs. Otherwise, they are easier to treat.

There is a type of tumor that forms in the stomach as a result of a conflict of hot and cold; first there is a sense of heat and consequent sweating, and then with even a little feeling of cold there is more pain associated with the tumor in the stomach. It is easy to identify because the stomach is as if tied in a knot, like a disease brought on by organisms in the stomach.

Then, there is a type of skin disorder that is very itchy with red spots on the skin. It is prevalent in India, and Tibetan medicine is effective against it. This disease occurs only in the skin; it comes from the blood's becoming filthy and from an increase in lymph. Due to diet and behavior, the patient's body is disturbed whereupon the illness manifests. A symptom of this is seemingly uncaused shivering. It can occur most anywhere on the body in red itchy spots with sharp points on the bumps. It is very itchy. When it dries in one place, it begins in another, etc.

Then, there is a joint tumor, the basic causes being those explained above. Mainly, it is a matter of the blood being disturbed by wind and improper diet and behavior. The principal joints where it forms are at the base of the neck, inside the neck, the skull joint at the temples, under the ears, and the jaw where the face joins the head. Pain is slight, and it is difficult to bring it to full ripeness — a small thing appears but does not fully develop; this makes it complicated. We put on a poultice externally and give medicines internally to cause the disease to come to a head; then a pus-like substance is drawn out. It is possible to mistake this sort of tumor for a swelling of sinusitis or with the earlier type of tumor that blocks the throat, the latter being in the flesh and this one being in the joint of the bone. There are eight varieties of this tumor: on the two sides of the skull, the two on the jaw, and several more connected with the neck. It is very easy to identify because the flesh, wherever it is, becomes like a white radish that has been frozen and allowed to thaw. It is very soft on the outside and harder on the inside.

Then, there is a tumor that appears on the fleshy part of the arms and legs; there are eight locations, the main being the forearms and the calves. The basic causation is as before. The pulse is very subtle and taut. The urine is the color of mustard seed oil. Pain is felt in the head. The patient shivers, developing goose bumps that in five minutes will disappear. The joints at the wrists and ankles will pain particularly. Sometimes, the person will vomit, have a blood-like diarrhea, and have muscle cramps at the onset of the disease. Sometimes also the timbre of the voice will change. The brilliance of the eyes and face will degenerate, and the person will speak crazily. Then, as the disease actually shows itself, the joints will swell.

There is another type of tumor that involves swelling all over the body. Sometimes the pain is greater, sometimes lesser. It is an unsteady disease in that sometimes the patient will get pain when hungry, sometimes when full; it is as if the disease is a liar. With regard to identifying this illness — before one is in the stage of the onset of the illness — prior to its appearance, the first vertebra, the cheeks, the middle of the back, and the area around the liver will become reddish. This is a sign that the disorder is about to enter the onset stage.

There is an earth variety of this tumor, which is hard and steady in size. The head of the swelling is dark. If it is a fire tumor, all of the swellings will have many small red spots on them. It will get big rapidly, and the edges will be as if burnt by fire. If it is associated with the water constituent, the body is as if cold; the head of the swelling has a blister, and lymph will come out of it. If it is associated with wind, the swelling will be whitish. It will fluctuate in size, changing at various times during the day.

Divisions of these tumors can be made by way of color. The white variety has a predominance of cold and has less pain; the pulse and urine will show signs of a cold disorder.

The black variety is more painful, and the pulse and urine show signs of an extreme heat disorder. Those of a mottled color are such that one day the urine is like a cold disorder, and then on another day it is like a hot disorder.

Then, there is also a wild tumor that quickly develops; a weaker form of the wild tumor stays the same size as when it first developed. There is also a variety in which the imperceptible organism mentioned earlier is very strong. Wherever this type of tumor is present there will be many bumps within that one swelling, like beads inside it. The "female" variety of the same disorder is small in size, and the pain is minimal. It is hard and unchanging.

I have condensed a number of headings because there are many, many subdivisions within them. I wonder if scientists in time will make a microscope that will be able to see the tiny organisms that are at the heart of these diseases.

Question: Are the organisms considered sentient beings?
Answer: Yes, they are atomic size sentient beings. As I said earlier, among the seven types, five can be seen by the eye, one with a microscope, and one probably cannot be seen even with a microscope.

There is another type of chronic sore or swelling, for which the causes and conditions in general are as explained before but the uncommon conditions giving rise to it are hard physical work and an increase of bad blood and lymph in the body. These swellings increase without the patient's knowledge, as if stealthily; then, wind brings these together in a mass. The mass is then together with organisms that are produced innately with the body whereupon chronic sores, which are extremely difficult to heal, form externally in the flesh, bone, and channels.

The symptoms of this disease when it is in the flesh are that the pulse is quick and quivering, the swelling is very hard, and the flesh is like a red radish and very messy under the surface. Regarding such a chronic sore on the bone, the signs are that the area of the bone at that place turns black and the pain is like a nail banged into that part of the bone. Regarding such a chronic sore in the veins, the sign is that the vein turns black, and it looks like an angry snake. These swellings are of various sizes: big, small, and so forth.

In the internal organs, these chronic sores are like tumors, very hard; for instance, if there is one on the small intestine, when you press on it, it will be very hard, and when it has ripened, pus will come out in the feces; therefore, care has to be taken.

There is one type of chronic sore that comes together with a contagious disease, passing from one person to another. It mainly comes from a bilious fever and occurs in the sinuses, brain, throat, kidneys, small intestine, lungs, stomach, and heart. It does not appear in the liver. Being bilious, the swelling is yellow; the person's face is yellow, the flesh turns yellow, the nails turn blue-black, and the patient shivers a lot. The pulse, when pressed, ceases; when you let go, it begins again. The urine is a mixture of yellow and red and is very viscous. The head and four primary joints — ankles and wrists — will ache. The patient will talk a lot but as if about to fall asleep. Especially, the underside of the tongue and the whites of the eyes under the flesh will be extremely yellow. No matter what is eaten the patient will have a bitter taste in the mouth. There is pain deep in the brain, and pus and blood come out of the nose.

If this type of disease forms in the lungs, the pain will be in the upper part of the body, and the mucus will be yellow. If it forms in the kidneys, the area around the kidneys will pain, and it will be difficult to defecate and urinate. If it forms in the stomach, the patient will have a bitter taste in the mouth and will vomit bile. If in the small intestines, the patient will have diarrhea and will defecate bile.

A contagious form of chronic swelling mainly forms in the throat, the inside of the mouth, and the sides of the neck. It is shaped like an egg. The basic causes and conditions are as before. If it pains a great deal, it is dangerous. There is a smaller one shaped like a half moon that pains only a little; it is less dangerous. Mostly, people mistake its initial stages for a knot in the channels and ignore it.

Another contagious one is call "many chronic swellings". The causes and conditions are as before. It involves one big swelling with lots of little ones around it. It could appear in the connective tissue behind the ears, in the armpits, breasts, thighs, groin, or backs of the knees. The pain will sometimes be greater, sometimes smaller, and the patient will have chills.

Another that is contagious is like earlier ones but has the additional feature that mainly it tends to form at the diaphragm. The external signs are difficult to notice, and it is not easy for it to ripen. Those afflicted with this are apt to get a pain when they lie down because stretching to one side or another will stretch the tumor.

Then there is another non-contagious type that occurs on the neck or higher up on the neck under the earlobes. One swelling appears, and then before this can heal, another one comes next to it, thereby circling the neck. An early symptom is that these begin to form under the earlobes on the neck, at which time the channels in the neck region will be uncomfortable. Once it circles the whole neck, it is difficult to treat. Different from other tumors, the medicines used to ripen tumors so that they can be drawn out will hardly ever work on this type.

That finishes this approach to the topic of tumors.

Question: Are all tumors curable?

Answer: Some are easy to cure; some are hard to cure; some can be cured, and some cannot; some are contagious; some are not. There are many divisions. The particular term here in this section "nyen" (*gnyan*) [translated in this latter section variously as "chronic sore" or "tumor"] refers to a swelling with abrasions whereas earlier the term "dren" (*skran*) [translated as "tumor"] referred to a lump.

Question: Are the contagious ones spread by touch?

Answer: You do not have to touch. If you stay with a person who has this problem, it could travel with the breath and so forth. The mode of contagion is similar to smallpox.

Question: Are all of the new diseases, the eighteen prophesied for a time later than when Buddha taught, tumors?
Answer: These eighteen do involve swelling; there are many, many divisions in each that I have skipped over. There are probably eighty different diseases under these eighteen categories. For instance, the one type that has male, female, and child varieties has sub-varieties in terms of wind, bile, and phlegm. Others have internal divisions according to the predominant element. I have identified these here only in a rough, condensed way.

Question: Are these classifications static or are they modified with time?
Answer: Those that are described in the text are for our era; thus, there is no need to change the descriptions. However, there are indeed clearer explanations in other books that one can consult.

Question: Does good diet make one free from these eighteen types of diseases?
Answer: There are diseases that come from one's own earlier actions, but the most important immediate factors are diet and behavior. In general, all diseases are instigated by the condition of improper eating or behavior. If one were able to eat and behave as is set forth by the Buddha, there would not be any reason to be sick during one's lifetime. One problem is that people nowadays eat many different sorts of things, even new combinations of substances; they smoke many different types of substances and drink many sorts of alcoholic drinks. Also, various types of fertilizers and so forth are being used to make vegetables grow more quickly and bigger, beyond their own nature. There is also the smoke and pollution that rises from new chemicals.

Question: Would you say that the use of chemical fertilizers is guaranteed to cause disease in the future?

Answer: I think that, for the most part, the use of fertilizers and so forth will create problems, especially for people who are not used to them, but certainly not for all. There is the further problem that the proper potency will not be in the particular food. They are physically bigger but not as tasty or as potent. In Tibet, vegetables were smaller but very delicious and potent. Here you have some that are very big but not potent or tasty.

For instance, because carrots are sweet, bugs attack them. In order to prevent that, scientists make fertilizers with substances in them that will keep away the bugs, but I think that this causes the sweetness of the carrots to go beyond their own measure; they become too sweet. This serves as a cause for there being so many cold disorders such as diabetes in the population nowadays.

Question: Sometimes there is criticism of Western medicine that it treats only the symptom and not the cause. Do you agree?

Answer: The important point is to get at the deeper causes. For instance, if there is water coming into your house and you keep trying to block it from inside, you cannot succeed; you ought to go outside, try to find out its source, and stop it from there.

Question: I assume that there are no hospitals in Tibet like those in the West. What do you think of going to a hospital for treatment?

Answer: One fact is that you are so much more prosperous than us and thus able to have and make use of such hospitals. Another factor is that our basic mode of thought is so very different from yours; we are mostly interested in practicing religion. Among our people there would be, out of one hundred, maybe one or two who were not interested in religion. That is where our main thought is directed. Our mode of thought seems to be opposite.

17 Virilification and Rejuvenation

Techniques of virilification are used to restore normal sexual functions.[172] Virilification refers to restoring or enhancing sexual performance and pleasure. It increases physical strength and promotes long life, and its importance lies in sustaining family lineages.

Virilification is mainly used for the male because if a male is unable to perform the sexual act, the family lineage cannot be sustained. Given that family lineages in Tibet were determined by the lineage of the father, the male was considered more important in this respect. A male implants the seed of birth, and when this seed, or semen, is infertile, then even though the male is surrounded by a hundred women, he cannot procreate.

Also, in terms of the practice of Secret Mantra, the same union of male and female is used with an entirely different consciousness. In this practice, the bliss arising from union of male and female is used to realize the emptiness of inherent existence in a totally non-dualistic and powerful way. For this practice to be effective, the regenerative fluid must be in good condition, and thus the importance of virilification is not limited to bringing physical pleasure or maintaining a family lineage but also includes enhancement of a high state of spiritual experience.

Before physicians can prescribe a means of virilification, they first must determine what is causing the deficiency in the patient's sexual life; they have to diagnose the cause of impotency or other sexual problem. This is done by examining the pulse and urine. From these methods of diagnosis, physicians can determine which of five types the disorder is: a wind, bile, phlegm, or blood disorder or a combination of any of these.

I will very briefly explain some of the symptoms of these five. If the cause of the semen disorder is wind, the semen has a blackish color, is rough, and has an astringent taste. If it is caused by a bile disorder, the semen is yellowish, has a sour taste, and gives off a bad odor as if rotten. In the case of a phlegm disorder, the semen is grayish-white, sweet in taste, very sticky, and cool. If it is caused by a blood disorder, the semen is putrid, having a decomposing nature.

If wind and phlegm together have created the order, the semen breaks very easily into particles. If blood and bile together have caused the disorder, the semen is pus-like. If bile and phlegm combine to cause the problem, the semen would be a knotty mass, not easily spreading. A wind and bile combination produces semen which is dry, without much fluid. If all four humors combine to cause the disorder, the semen has the characteristics of the patient's urine, cloudy and as if rotten.

The main aim of a physician in treating such a patient is to remove any of these causes, thereby restoring the semen to a natural, fertile condition. Also, in the case of females, the menstrual blood is to be examined similarly in terms of these same five factors — wind, bile, phlegm, blood, and combinations.

Fertile, faultless semen is white, sweet, and heavy; it should have the qualities of taste similar to those of honey. In the case of a female, to be fertile the color of the menstrual blood should be like the blood of a mountain rabbit.

Fertile semen and menstrual blood — if it drops on a piece of cloth — can be easily washed, whereas in the case of the infertile, it cannot be easily removed.

The main way to treat patients with sexual disorders such as infertility and impotency is to restore the power of the kidneys and to increase the amount of semen. The treatment is in the form of oral medications or lotions applied at the genitals.

With regard to the medicinal ingredients for virilification, in Tibet there is a white snow frog, the flesh of which acts as a powerful sexual stimulant. It is the principal ingredient in virilification medicines, others being herbal. It is important to remove the toxins in the frog flesh by a process of removal, leaving only the part that does not harm. This frog might sound fictitious, but I had an uncle who said that the flesh of this frog was eaten by several inhabitants of his area, who became seriously ill because of the toxins.

Apart from medication, the Tibetan text speaks of environmental factors of pleasant sights, sounds, odors, touches, and tastes for heightening sexual pleasure, and it also describes the nature of the partner in terms of age, physical appearance, and so forth. Such sources of pleasure act as means of virilification, thereby sustaining the family lineage.

In conclusion, the reasons for virilification are, as mentioned earlier, twofold: non-spiritual and spiritual. The aim of the non-spiritual is to sustain family lineages particularly of higher classes who, in Tibet, had great responsibilities to support religious practice; it also is used frequently to restore proper sexual functioning. Regarding the spiritual, it was mentioned earlier that the highest purpose of virilification is to enhance experience of the bliss of union so that the bliss consciousness can be used to realize the nature of phenomena, their emptiness of inherent existence, in a particularly powerful way in order that obstructions to the altruistic state of Buddhahood can be overcome quickly.

REJUVENATION

The treatment of aging is called essence-extraction.[173]
According to the Four Tantras, from the time of birth up to
age sixteen, one is a child; from age sixteen to seventy, one
is an adult; from seventy on, one is old.

The old have a predominance of wind humor. Because of
this predominance of wind, when one gets to be about sixty,
one needs to engage in techniques to overcome wind. For
instance, you should eat special foods in accordance with
your constitution. Moreover, if your own nature is predominantly wind, you should emphasize the drinking of
meat broth, bone broth, and milk. If you have a predominance of bile, you should eat more new butter, new yogurt,
and take bone broth of freshly killed goat or sheep. If you
have a predominance of phlegm, you should eat more old
butter and drink broth made from aged lamb — lamb that
has been allowed to age. In addition, you should take a
medicine called "essence-extraction" for rejuvenation.

The text explains this latter topic in terms of its benefit,
the mode of procedure of the religious rite that is involved,
the place for performing the rite, and the basis, that is, the
body of the person who is practicing the rite. The benefit of
performing this rite, which involves taking the essence-
extraction medicine, is that you come to have longer life,
you do not grow old so easily, it makes you younger,
increases digestive fire and the strength of the body, makes
the senses and memory clearer, makes your mind sharper,
yields a resonant voice, and makes you more virile.

The place of performance should be clean and isolated in
the sense of being quiet and not in the midst of commotion
such as in a busy city, being pleasant to yourself, and
having all of the concordant circumstances for remaining
there; you should be free of interference, for you have to
conduct the rite without interruption. You perform the rite,
take the medicine, and imagine the descent of ambrosia into
yourself; thus, it would interfere if there were interrup-

tions. The practitioner should not be extremely old, because if so, there would no longer be any point in the practice.

During the practice, you should not over-expose yourself to heat from fire or to the sun, or generate a lot of desire, or work very hard physically or mentally. You should not eat any rotten foods and should give up eating sour foods as well as raw foods. You should not take a lot of salt. Then, at a time when the planets and stars are in an auspicious position, you should wash your body — washing with lentil powder or soap and then rubbing on oil. That is external bathing. Internal bathing is done by way of a medicine that is compounded of nine substances, which are mixed with cow urine; it is taken in the form of a pill or with cow urine. The special qualities of cow urine are that it cleans the lymph and blood in the body. If, without doing internal and external cleaning, you engaged in the practice of essence-extraction for rejuvenation and virilification, it would be like trying to dye a cloth that was soiled — the dye would not take in the places that were soiled. When bathing is performed, subsequent practice of essence-extraction is supremely successful.

The medicine is processed in an unusual way; it is not like the usual procedure of making pills, but resembles the way that we make vitamins. All types of essence-extract medicines are made in a process of boiling various substances and then, in series, adding milk, boiling it down, and adding butter, boiling that down. Finally, you get to the point where even though it is boiling you can stick your finger in the mixture but it does not hurt; you can sprinkle it in the fire, and it will not even sizzle. Changes have been brought about in the substances. A powdered sugar and dried honey are added, and finally the pill is rolled. I am summarizing a complicated procedure.

You take the medicine for, at the most, six months; the average is two to three months. A form compounded of five metallic substances is the supreme of medicines to increase life span for a person with a predominance of blood and bile. There is another type composed of another set of five substances using honey for those who have a predominance of phlegm and cold; it increases the life span, develops more flesh, and ignites the inner digestive fire. There is another version that has the three fruits in it; it causes your sense faculties to become clearer, generates strength, clears away sicknesses which are triple combinations of the humors, and sets you in a younger state. Then there is another version made from fluids drawn from flowers; the signs of old age disappear; you come to have the body of a sixteen-year-old, the dexterity of a lion, the power of an elephant, the brilliant color of a peacock, the swiftness of a horse, and a life span like that of the sun and moon. There are nine varieties of the medicine.

The main part of the ritual is meditation and repetition of mantra. Practitioners generate [or imagine] themselves as a deity and the medicine as a deity. Meditating on the medicine as a deity, the meditator then imagines that it melts into light and turns into ambrosia. This is a *medicinal* ambrosia of freedom from sickness, a *wisdom* ambrosia of non-degeneration, and a *life* ambrosia of immortality. If done properly, the medicine will have the effects described.

In Tibet, there were many accounts of people who succeeded at this practice; even though old, they became young again, living even a hundred thirty or a hundred fifty years. Nowadays, there is one ge-shay [high level scholar] in Hla-sa whose body became younger through this practice; he lives without eating coarse food, merely taking this medicine. When the Chinese took over our country, they decided to test him by putting him in a room for fifteen days with no food except for this essence-extract. He remained fine, meditating. The Chinese were impressed and left him alone; they said, "You are a true practitioner." However, his skin tone is not good because he does not eat any butter, meat, and so forth. Every day he probably takes the medicine three times — a large pill [about the size of a bubble gum ball] each time.

A person with a predominance of wind should take a form of essence-extract the potency of which is heavy. A person with a predominance of bile should take one the potency of which is cool, and a person with predominant phlegm should take one which is rough.

Many in Tibet took the version that is only a flower extract; there also were many who lived for a year or two on just one type of essence-extract. If that ge-shay were able to take the flower extract version, his skin tone would improve.

If it is manufactured well and the person does the meditation well, signs of success emerge: the body becomes younger; white hair turns black again, and even new teeth can come in. When such signs appear, you have succeeded, and it is not necessary to take more. However, if in future years you did take more, you would improve even more.

Even if you cannot bring together all the concordant circumstances for this practice, it will still be beneficial; you will live longer. If while engaged in this practice, some other illness attacks, you should get rid of that other illness before continuing. Once that illness is cured, you can return to the practice.

A reincarnation of Ma-ji-lap-drön lived to be one hundred and eighty; it has been only about twenty-five years since her death. She used a type of essence-extract that is taken with food. I met her a number of times.

18 Meditative Transformation of Medicine

In general, Shākyamuni Buddha taught doctrines in accordance with the predispositions and interests of trainees; among these doctrines, the science of medicine is particularly supreme. The reason for this is that, for instance, ordinarily the six perfections of giving, ethics, patience, effort, concentration, and wisdom cannot immediately be practiced simultaneously and instead are practiced one by one, but, with medicine, once its essentials have been realized and put into practice, the six perfections are accomplished simultaneously.

From among the three forms of the perfection of giving — giving things, non-fright, and doctrine — the giving of medicine itself is a giving of material things. Advice that calms the patient, thereby restoring a relaxed attitude, is a giving of non-fright, relief from anxiety, as is the giving of medicine that protects life. Also, advice to patients to repeat mantra and engage in religious activities is a giving of doctrine. In addition, since the medicines are blessed into a magnificent state through being implanted with mantra, such giving is associated with doctrine. Similarly, treatment of the poor without fee fulfills the practice of the giving of things, the giving of non-fright, and the giving of doctrine.

With respect to ethics, physicians' maintenance of medicinal ingredients and medicines themselves in their proper, clean environment without improperly mixing them together fulfills the practice of ethics, as does their emphasis on others' welfare rather than their own. With respect to patience, when physician-pharmacologists go to the mountains, for instance, to collect herbs and so forth, their hands can be cut by sharp leaves and pierced by thorns; they become weary from the long hiking and hard work. Their patience, their forbearance, fulfills the practice of patience.

Similarly, their performing with great effort what needs to be done in making medicines at the appropriate time during the seasons — not putting it off to later — fulfills the practice of effort. Furthermore, the practice of concentration is fulfilled through deeds of meditation and mantra as I will explain below. Also, physicians' detailed understanding of the qualities, tastes, potencies, and reasons for these due to predominance of the elements fulfills the practice of wisdom. In this way, the practice of medicine should be suffused with practice of the six perfections.

About the practice of concentration, Buddhist medicine is not like non-Buddhist medicine, for it utilizes three levels of potency — the entities of medicinal ingredients, the power of mantra, and the power of meditative stabilization. The ingredients basically may be the same, but in the Buddhist system various medicines are activated through the practice of specific deities. There are many types of meditative activation of medicines relative to various deities; for instance, the deity Hayagrīva is used for medicines counteracting contagious diseases. First, the physician gathers all the ingredients to manufacture the medicine; a ritual is done before the ingredients are made into the medicine and then again after the pills have been made. In these rituals, the physician, or a lama, meditatively imagines himself or herself to be Hayagrīva and also imagines the pills to be Hayagrīvas. The two, oneself as Hayagrīva and the pills as Hayagrīva, are considered to be fused as one undifferentiable entity. Because the deities and mantras used in the rituals differ depending on the purpose, the potentializing effects on the medicines differ.

With regard to the general structure of the ritual, whether the pills are put in a begging bowl or not, they are imagined to be so by the lama, who first takes refuge in the Buddha, the Doctrine, and the Spiritual Community and then generates an altruistic intention to become enlightened. After that, the lama/physician dissolves into the emptiness of inherent existence, re-emerging as Hayagrīva or Bhaiṣhajyaguru, with a complete mandala, if done extensively, and otherwise alone. Bhaiṣhajyaguru is blue in color like the sky; his body is clear when looking from the outside and clear when looking outward from inside. His right hand makes the gesture of meditative equipoise; his left hand holds a begging bowl filled with ambrosia. A similar King of Physicians is meditated also in front of yourself. Then, you — as Bhaiṣhajyaguru — invite in all the Buddhas of the ten directions as Kings Of Physicians[174] who dissolve into yourself and the deity in front. At this point, you think that you have become the actual entity of the King Of Physicians. Rays of light are emitted from the King Of Physicians in front, gathering medicinal and nutritional essences from the ten directions and withdrawing them into the medicine in the begging bowl, into which they dissolve. Then, mantra is repeated.

While repeating mantra, you keep your body in the seven-featured posture of Vairochana. Your feet are in the adamantine cross-legged posture; your hands are as indicated above, or both hands are arranged in the gesture of meditative equipoise with the right hand on top of the left and the two thumbs touching; your eyes are aimed at the point of the nose; your backbone is straight like an arrow; your neck is slightly bent like that of a peacock; your shoulders are level, not leaning to one side or the other; your tongue touches the ridge behind the upper teeth. Once your body is set this way, you imagine that at your heart is a flat moon disc with an *om* standing on top of it. The syllable *om* emits light rays filling the ten directions; from these rays of light goddesses of offering emerge, making offerings to all the Buddhas. After that, the goddesses, together with the Buddhas' qualities of exalted body, speech, and mind dissolve into the rays of light which are withdrawn into your own heart and dissolve into your own continuum. The qualities of exalted body return as white light rays that dissolve into the crown of your own head; the qualities of exalted speech return as red light rays that dissolve into your neck, and the qualities of exalted mind return as blue light rays that dissolve into your heart.

Again, light rays are emitted from your heart; these strike all six types of sentient beings — hell-beings, hungry ghosts, animals, humans, demigods, and gods — entering their bodies and minds, thereby relieving them of their particular sufferings. In general, gods suffer from extreme grief when they are about to die, from the realization that they will be reborn in a lower state; demigods suffer from jealousy and consequent fighting with the gods; humans suffer from birth, aging, sickness, and death; animals suffer from stupidity and being used for others' purposes; hungry ghosts suffer from hunger and thirst; and hell-beings suffer from heat and cold. The rays of light relieve each of these beings in appropriate form.

Similarly, you imagine that light rays spread out from the heart of the King Of Physicians in front of you, radiating in the ten directions, entering into the four elements, and turning them into highly potentialized medicines. These light rays return and dissolve into the medicines in Bhaishajyaguru's begging bowl. This is how the power of mantra and meditative stabilization affects the potencies of medicines.

The King Of Physicians is also called the Supreme

Physician;[175] "medicine" has the sense of helping, and "lama" means that of which there is nothing higher. Ordinary doctors are indeed physicians,[176] but they are not Supreme Physicians — omniscient physicians — whereas Bhaishajyaguru is. Bhaiṣhajyaguru has eradicated all desire, hatred, and ignorance in his continuum as well as their fruits — wind, bile, and phlegm — and can assist others in doing the same; hence, he is a King Of Physicians.

Since he knows the dispositions and interests of each and every sentient being, he can speak doctrine that accords with their situation; therefore, it is said that through only hearing his name, the sufferings of bad transmigrations are cleared away. If that is the case, then it need not be mentioned that repeating his mantra is very beneficial. Even great heaps of gold and silver cannot keep beings from being reborn in bad transmigrations; thus, it is very worthwhile to assume the meditative posture, imagine yourself as the actual King Of Physicians, and with one-pointed concentration recite his mantra. Otherwise, you can imagine the King Of Physicians in front of yourself in imagination. In either case, look carefully at the blue color of his body, how he is sitting, the shape of his eyes, the gesture that his hands are displaying, and so forth. Also, think about his qualities and altruistic activities, and within such reflection repeat his mantra:

Namo bhagavate bhaiṣhajya-guru-vaiḍūrya-prabhā-rājāya tathāgatāyārhate samyak-saṃbuddhāya tad yathā: oṃ bhaiṣhajye bhaiṣhajye bhaiṣhajya-rājā-samudgate svāhā.[177]

Appendix 1
Lists

Three humors
  wind (air)
  bile
  phlegm

Three poisons
  desire
  hatred
  obscuration

Four Tantras
  Root Tantra
  Explanatory Tantra
  Oral Tradition Tantra
  Last Tantra

Five biles
  1. digestive bile
  2. color-regulating bile
  3. determining bile
  4. sight bile
  5. complexion-clearing

Five phlegms
1. supportive phlegm
2. decomposing phlegm
3. experiencing phlegm
4. satisfying phlegm
5. connective phlegm

Five winds
1. life-sustaining wind
2. ascending wind
3. pervasive wind
4. fire-accompanying wind
5. descending wind

Five vital organs
heart
lungs
liver
spleen
kidneys

Seven physical constituents
1. nutritional essence
2. blood
3. flesh
4. fat
5. bone
6. marrow
7. regenerative fluid

Six reservoir organs
stomach
small intestine
large intestine
gall bladder
seminal vesicle
urinary bladder

Three excretions
1. feces
2. urine
3. perspiration

Appendix 2
Outline of *The Ambrosia Heart Tantra*

By Dr. Yeshi Donden
Translated by Ven. Jhampa Kelsang (Alan Wallace)

(Dr. Donden's book was published by the Library of Tibetan Works and Archives, Dharmsala, India, without an index; therefore, a more detailed table of contents is provided here; the numbers after the entries refer to page numbers in the book. *The Ambrosia Heart Tantra* is available from the Library of Tibetan Works and Archives and from Snow Lion Publications.)

Bibliography

(For more extensive bibliographies on Tibetan medicine, see the entries under Finckh, Tsarong, Clifford, and Badjajew.)

Avedon, John. *In Exile From the Land of Snows*. New York: Knopf, 1979.

Badjajew, Peter, Jr., Badmajew, Vladimir, Jr., and Park, Lynn. *Healing Herbs: The Heart Of Tibetan Medicine*. Berkeley: Red Lotus Press, 1982.

Birnbaum, Raoul. *The Healing Buddha*. Boulder: Shambhala, 1979.

Clifford, Terry. *Tibetan Buddhist Medicine And Psychiatry*. York Beach, Maine: Samuel Weiser, 1984.

Das, Sarat Chandra. *A Tibetan-English Dictionary with Sanskrit Synonyms*. Calcutta, 1902.

Day-śi-śang-gyay-gya-tso (*sangs rgyas rgya mtsho, sde srid*, 1653-1705). *Bai ḍūr sṅon po*, vols. 1-4. Leh: T.Y. Tashigangpa, 1973. Smanrtsis Shesrig Spendzod Series vols. 51-4.

Donden, Dr. Yeshi. "Pulse Diagnosis in Tibetan Medicine: Translated from the first chapter of the fourth Tantra". *Tibetan Medicine*, Series No.1, 1980, pp.13-29.

Donden, Dr. Yeshi. *The Ambrosia Heart Tantra*, vol. 1. Trans. Jhampa Kelsang (Alan Wallace). Dharmasala: Library of Tibetan Works and Archives, 1977.

Emmerick, R.E. "A Chapter From The *Rgyud-bźi*". *Asia Major*, vol. xix, part 2, pp.141-162.

Emmerick, R.E. "Some Lexical Items From The *Rgyud-bźi*". *Proceedings Of The Csoma De Kŏrös Memorial Symposium.* Ed. Louis Ligeti. Budapest: Akadémiai Kiadó, 1978.

Finckh, Elisabeth. *Foundations Of Tibetan Medicine,* vol. 1. Trans. by Fredericka M. Houser. London: Watkins, 1978.

Goldstein, Melvyn C. *English-Tibetan Dictionary Of Modern Tibetan.* Berkeley: U. Cal. Press, 1984.

Goldstein, Melvyn C. *Tibetan-English Dictionary Of Modern Tibetan.* Kathmandu: Ratna Pustak Bhandar, 1975.

Hopkins, Jeffrey. *Meditation on Emptiness.* London: Wisdom Publications, 1983.

Jam-bel-dor-jay (*'jam dpal rdo rje*). *An Illustrated Tibeto-Mongolian Materia Medica Of Ayurveda of 'jam-dpal-rdo-rje Of Mongolia.* Ed. Lokesh Chandra. New Delhi: International Academy of Indian Culture, 1971. Śata-piṭaka series, Indo-Asian Literatures, vol. 82.

Norbu, Namkhai. *On Birth And Life: A Treatise On Tibetan Medicine.* English trans. Dr. Barry Simmons. Italy: Tipografia Commerciale Venezia, 1983.

Rabgay, Lobsang. "Pulse Analysis in Tibetan Medicine". *Tibetan Medicine,* Series No. 3, 1981, pp.45-52. Dharamsala: Library of Tibetan Works and Archives.

Rabgay, Lobsang. "Urine Analysis in Tibetan Medicine". *Tibetan Medicine,* Series No. 3, 1981, pp.53-60. Dharamsala: Library of Tibetan Works and Archives.

Rechung Rinpoche. *Tibetan Medicine Illustrated In Original Texts.* London: 1973. Rpt. as *Tibetan Medicine.* Berkeley: U. of California Press, 1976.

Tsarong, T.J., trans. and ed. *Fundamentals Of Tibetan Medicine.* Dharamsala: Tibetan Medical Centre, 1981.

Vogel, Claus. *Vāgbhaṭa's Aṣṭāṅgahṛdayasaṃhitā, The First Five Chapters Of Its Tibetan Version.* Wiesbaden, 1965.

Wylie, Turrell. "A Standard System of Tibetan Transcription". *Harvard Journal of Asiatic Studies,* Vol. 22, 1959, pp.261-7.

Notes

1. This section is drawn from John Avedon's marvelous book *In Exile From the Land of Snows* (New York: Knopf, 1979). See pages 137-56 for more of Dr. Donden's fascinating story. Elisabeth Finckh, in her *Foundations Of Tibetan Medicine*, vol. 1, trans. by Fredericka M. Houser (London: Watkins, 1978), p.25, identifies the village as near Lake Yar-drok (*yar 'brog*).

2. *mkhyen rab nor bu*, 1882-1962. See Elisabeth Finckh, *Foundations Of Tibetan Medicine*, vol. 1, p.30, for three books written by Kyen-rap-nor-bu (items 13, 14, and 15).

3. *rlung, mkhris pa, bad kan*. As mentioned in the Preface, these terms have very wide meanings that are not limited to our usual contemporary notions of wind (air), bile, and phlegm. These are the three *nyes pa* (*dosha*), which literally means "faults", most likely because they can give rise to all sorts of problems; here *nyes pa* has been translated loosely as "humor" since this is more familiar. Nevertheless, strictly speaking, the "humors" are *fluids* as in the four elemental fluids of the body — blood, phlegm, black bile, and yellow bile — in other systems.

4. *rgyud bzhi*. The longer title of this work is *bdud rtsi snying po yan lag brgyad pa gsang ba man ngag gi rgyud*. For an excellent overview of the medical literature, see Elisabeth Finckh, *Foundations Of Tibetan Medicine*, vol.1, chapters four and five, pp.27-39.

5. *rtsa ba'i rgyud*.

6. *bshad pa'i rgyud*.

7. *man ngag gi rgyud.*

8. *phyi ma'i rgyud.*

9. For an overview of the Four Tantras, see Elisabeth Finckh, *Foundations Of Tibetan Medicine,* vol.1, chapter five, pp.31-39; and T.J. Tsarong, trans. and ed., *Fundamentals Of Tibetan Medicine* (Dharamsala: Tibetan Medicine Centre, 1981), pp.100-108.

10. For other presentations, see Elisabeth Finckh, *Foundations Of Tibetan Medicine,* vol. 1, chapters six and seven, pp.41-77; Dr. Yeshi Donden, *The Ambrosia Heart Tantra,* vol. 1, trans. Jhampa Kelsang (Alan Wallace), (Dharmasala: Library of Tibetan Works and Archives, 1977), pp.41-42; R.E. Emmerick, A Chapter From The *Rgyud-bźi, Asia Major,* vol. xix, part 2, pp.141-162; and T.J. Tsarong, trans. and ed., *Fundamentals Of Tibetan Medicine,* pp.45-70.

11. *gnas lugs rtsa ba.* The word *gnas lugs* has the sense of "status" or "actual situation". This root is also called the *gnas lugs nad gzhi,* the "actual situation [of the body] which is the basis of disease".

12. Not only are the three humors similar to the Sāṃkhya presentation of three qualities (*yon tan gsum, triguṇa*) of *sattva, rajas,* and *tamas* but also the terms for a balanced state (*rnam par ma gyur pa*) and an unbalanced state (*rnam par gyur pa*) are similar. In Highest Yoga Tantra, the three subtler consciousnesses preceding the mind of clear light are called *sattva, rajas,* and *tamas* in Dzong-ka-ba's *Great Exposition Of Secret Mantra.*

13. For the Sanskrit and variations of the Tibetan for the five winds, five biles, and five phlegms, see R.E. Emmerick, "A Chapter From The *Rgyud-bźi*", *Asia Major,* vol. xix, part 2, p.148-150.

14. See Dr. Yeshi Donden, *The Ambrosia Heart Tantra,* vol. 1, pp.33-35 and Elisabeth Finckh, *Foundations Of Tibetan Medicine,* vol. 1, pp.59-68, 77.

15. Classification of diseases is also done by way of physical basis into five types: disorders specific to males, to females, to children, to the aged, and those common to all. See *The Ambrosia Heart Tantra,* vol. 1, pp.87-110. Also, another mode of division of diseases is by way of characteristics; this is mentioned briefly in *The Ambrosia Heart Tantra,* vol. 1, pp.110.

16. The corresponding section in *The Ambrosia Heart Tantra* is on pp.76-77.

17. The corresponding section in *The Ambrosia Heart Tantra* is on pp.78-80.

18. The corresponding section in *The Ambrosia Heart Tantra* is on p.81.

19. For a list of organs, see Appendix 1, pp.220-221.

20. For discussion of textual difficulties, etc., with the "fifteen paths of circulation", see R.E. Emmerick, "A Chapter From The *Rgyud-bźi*", *Asia Major*, vol. xix, part 2, pp.154-155, which is cited in Elisabeth Finckh, *Foundations Of Tibetan Medicine*, vol. 1, pp.90-92, n.8a.

21. The Library of Tibetan Works and Archives, Dharamsala, India, publishes a magazine called *Tibetan Medicine* that is very helpful on a wide range of topics. Articles on pulse are to be found in Series No. 1, 1980, pp.13-29, and Series No. 3, 1981, pp.45-52; the former is "Pulse Diagnosis in Tibetan Medicine: Translated from the first chapter of the fourth Tantra", by Yeshi Donden through Sonam Topgay, and the latter is "Pulse Analysis in Tibetan Medicine", by Lobsang Rabgay. Sonam Topgay and Lobsang Rabgay are the same person.

In Day-śi-śang-gyay-gya-tso's *Blue Vaiḍūrya*, Vol. 4, the section on pulse is pp.2-84. "Vaiḍūrya" has been variously identified as lapis lazuli, cat'seye, and beryl; for a brief discussion see Elisabeth Finckh, *Foundations Of Tibetan Medicine*, vol. 1, pp.88 n.3.

22. In Day-śi-śang-gyay-gya-tso's *Blue Vaiḍūrya*, Vol. 4, the section on prerequisites begins at 32.2.

23. In Day-śi-śang-gyay-gya-tso's *Blue Vaiḍūrya*, Vol. 4, the corresponding section begins at 33.4.

24. In Day-śi-śang-gyay-gya-tso's *Blue Vaiḍūrya*, Vol. 4, the corresponding section begins at 34.6.

25. Technically, the distance is the length of the second phalanx of the thumb.

26. In Day-śi-śang-gyay-gya-tso's *Blue Vaiḍūrya*, Vol. 4 the corresponding section begins at 37.4.

27. In Day-śi-śang-gyay-gya-tso's *Blue Vaiḍūrya*, Vol. 4, the corresponding section begins at 38.1.

28. In Day-śi-śang-gyay-gya-tso's *Blue Vaiḍūrya*, Vol. 4, the corresponding section begins at 40.1.

29. In Day-śi-śang-gyay-gya-tso's *Blue Vaiḍūrya*, Vol. 4, the corresponding section begins at 42.4.

30. In Day-ŝi-ŝang-gyay-gya-tso's *Blue Vaidūrya*, Vol. 4, the corresponding section begins at 48.1.

31. *klu srin.*

32. *dam sri.*

33. In Day-ŝi-ŝang-gyay-gya-tso's *Blue Vaidūrya*, Vol. 4, the corresponding section begins at 62.5.

34. In Day-ŝi-ŝang-gyay-gya-tso's *Blue Vaidūrya*, Vol. 4, the corresponding section begins at 66.3.

35. For a list of organs, see Appendix 1, pp.220-221.

36. In Day-ŝi-ŝang-gyay-gya-tso's *Blue Vaidūrya*, Vol. 4, the corresponding section begins at 74.4.

37. In Day-ŝi-ŝang-gyay-gya-tso's *Blue Vaidūrya*, Vol. 4, the corresponding section begins at 78.4.

38. *lha srung.*

39. *rgyal po.*

40. *klu bdud.*

41. *klu btsan.*

42. *sa bdag.*

43. *gre mo.*

44. *gre po gnyan.*

45. *gnyan.*

46. *mtsho sman.*

47. *glu bsen mo.*

48. *bkor bdag rgyal po.*

49. *btsan.*

50. *bdud glu btsan.*

51. *ma mo byang sman.*

52. *glu gyan.*

53. *sa bdag.*

54. In Day-ŝi-ŝang-gyay-gya-tso's *Blue Vaidūrya*, Vol. 4, the corresponding section begins at 80.3.

55. *chos mngon pa'i mdzod, abhidharmakosha.*

56. For a similar presentation by Lobsang Rabgay, see his article "Urine Analysis in Tibetan Medicine" in *Tibetan Medicine*, Series No. 3, 1981, pp.53-60, published by the Library of Tibetan Works and Archives, Dharamsala, India. In Day-ŝi-ŝang-gyay-gya-tso's *Blue Vaidūrya*, Vol. 4, the section on urinalysis is pp.84-127.

57. In Day-ŝi-ŝang-gyay-gya-tso's *Blue Vaidūrya*, Vol. 1, the corresponding section begins at 308.2. See also *The Ambrosia*

Heart Tantra, pp.112-116.

58. In Day-śi-śang-gyay-gya-tso's *Blue Vaiḍūrya*, Vol. 1, the corresponding section begins at 322.2. See also *The Ambrosia Heart Tantra*, pp.117-119.

59. In Day-śi-śang-gyay-gya-tso's *Blue Vaiḍūrya*, Vol. 1, the corresponding section begins at 332.2. See also *The Ambrosia Heart Tantra*, pp.120-122.

60. In Day-śi-śang-gyay-gya-tso's *Blue Vaiḍûrya*, Vol. 1, the section on diet begins at 336.4, page 336 being misnumbered as 340. The order of these pages in the Leh 1973 edition is confused; 339=335, 340=336, 335=337, 336=338, 337=339, and 338=340.

61. *khra ma.*

62. *so ba.*

63. *sre da.* In Day-śi-śang-gyay-gya-tso's *Blue Vaiḍūrya*, Vol. 1, 337.6, read *sre da* for *sra da* in accordance with 339.1.

64. *rgya sran.* Goldstein identifies this as "broad bean" in his *English-Tibetan Dictionary Of Modern Tibetan* (Berkeley: U. Cal. Press, 1984), p.42, but as "lentil" in his *Tibetan-English Dictionary Of Modern Tibetan* (Kathmandu: Ratna Pustak Bhandar, 1975), p.266.

65. *ma sha.*

66. *sran chung leb mo.*

67. *til dkar nag.*

68. *zar ma.*

69. *bra bo.*

70. In Day-śi-śang-gyay-gya-tso's *Blue Vaiḍūrya*, Vol. 1, the section on animals begins at 340.2, page 340 being misnumbered as 338.

71. *rma bya.*

72. *gong mo.*

73. *sreg pa.*

74. *skyung ka.*

75. *bya nag.*

76. *ne tso.*

77. *khu byug.*

78. *thi ba zhar ma.*

79. *skya ga.*

80. *'jol mo*, Pomatorhinus swinhoei.

81. *byi'u.*

82. *sha ba.*
83. *gla ba.*
84. *dgo ba,* Procapra pictaudata.
85. *gnyan.*
86. *ri bong.*
87. *brtsod.*
88. *gna' ba.*
89. *rgya.* In Das's *Tibetan-English Dictionary* (p. 303) this is identified as "animals of the deer class, in appearance like the *Nilgai,* possibly the saiga-antelope."
90. *kha sha.*
91. *ra rgod.*
92. *phag rgod.*
93. *ma he.*
94. *bse ru.*
95. *smyug stag.*
96. *rkyang.*
97. *g.yak rgod/ 'brong.*
98. *mdzo rgod.*
99. *stag.*
100. *gzig.*
101. *dom.*
102. *dred.*
103. *gsa'.*
104. *spyang kyi.*
105. *g.yi.*
106. *wa.*
107. *'phar ba.*
108. *sbre.* In Das's *Tibetan-English Dictionary* (p. 944) this is identified as a weasel or a stone-fox.
109. *bya rgod.*
110. *khva ta.*
111. *bya rlag.*
112. *ne le, 'ol pa.* In Das's *Tibetan-English Dictionary* the *ne le* (p. 743) is identified as the harrier-hawk; Das also refers to an identification as the kite, but the *'ol pa* which Day-si-sang-gyay-gya-tso's *Blue Vaidūrya,* Vol. 1, (341.1) gives as a gloss for *ne le* is identified by Das (p.1120) as the kite.
113. *bya rog.*
114. *'ug pa.*

115. *khra.*
116. *mdzo.*
117. *'bri.*
118. *g.yak.*
119. *'bri.*
120. *rnga mo.*
121. *rta.*
122. *bong bu.*
123. *ba lang.*
124. *skom po.*
125. *ra.*
126. *lug.*
127. *khyi.*
128. *phag pa.*
129. *khyim bya.*
130. *byi la, zhi mi.*
131. *'phyi ba.*
132. *gzugs mo byi thur.*
133. *sbal pa.*
134. *sbrul.*
135. *grum pa.*
136. *rmigs pa.*
137. *rtsangs pa.*
138. *sdig pa.*
139. *khrung khrung.* In Das's *Tibetan-English Dictionary* (p. 172) this also is identified as "the stork".
140. *ngang skya.*
141. *ngur pa.*
142. *so bya, so to rog po.*
143. *skyar mo.*
144. *sram.*
145. *nya.*
146. *'brum nag.*
147. In Day-śi-śang-gyay-gya-tso's *Blue Vaiḍūrya*, Vol. 1, the section on oils begins at 344.4
148. In Day-śi-śang-gyay-gya-tso's *Blue Vaiḍūrya*, Vol. 1, the section on herbs begins at 346.6.
149. *lcum*, Rheum palmatum or Rheum emodi.
150. *chu lo*, similar to Rheum nobile.
151. In Day-śi-śang-gyay-gya-tso's *Blue Vaiḍūrya*, Vol. 1, the

section on cooking begins at 348.1.

152. *kheng po*. For speculation on the meaning of this term and others, see R.E. Emmerick, "Some Lexical Items From The *Rgyud-bźi*", *Proceedings Of The Csoma De Körös Memorial Symposium*, Ed. Louis Ligeti (Budapest: Akadémiai Kiadó, 1978. On p.105, Emmerick suggests "puffed up" for *kheng po*, based on the basic meaning of *khengs pa* as "puffed up, proud, haughty, arrogant".

153. *lcam pa*.

154. *pe khur*, glossed as *tha ram* in Day-śi-śang-gyay-gya-tso's *Blue Vaiḍūrya*, Vol. 1, p.350.2; also Plantago depressa.

155. *dva ba*, either Arisaema intermedium or Typhonium giganteum.

156. *sne'u*.

157. *mon sne dmar po*.

158. *lo gsar me tog*.

159. *skyabs*.

160. *khur mang*.

161. *sngo sga*, Cremanthodium.

162. *lca ba*. This is identified as "a sort of carrot" in Das's *Tibetan-English Dictionary*, p.396.

163. *ra mnye*, Polygonatum cirrhifolium.

164. *la phug*.

165. *sgog skya* and *sgog sngon*, identified in Das's *Tibetan-English Dictionary*, p.326, as *Allium nival Jacqm.* and *Allium rubellum*.

166. *g.yer ma*, zanthoxlyum tibetanum. This is identified in Das's *Tibetan-English Dictionary*, p.1155, as *Capsicum*.

167. *sga*.

168. *shing kun*.

169. In Day-śi-śang-gyay-gya-tso's *Blue Vaiḍūrya*, Vol. 1, the section on drink begins at 351.2.

170. *gcin snyi*. In Day-śi-śang-gyay-gya-tso's *Blue Vaiḍūrya*, Vol. 2, this section begins at 519.2. This chapter is based on a lecture that was given at the University of Virginia Medical School.

171. *zangs ltar dmar ba*.

172. In Day-śi-śang-gyay-gya-tso's *Blue Vaiḍūrya*, Vol. 3, the section on virilification (*ro tsa ba*) begins on 510.6.

173. *bcud len*. In Day-śi-śang-gyay-gya-tso's *Blue*

Vaiḍūrya, Vol. 3, the section on rejuvenation begins on 496.6.

174. *sman pa'i rgyal po.*
175. *sman bla, bhaiṣhajyaguru.*
176. *sman pa.*
177. The mantra as it appears here differs only slightly from that cited by Raoul Birnbaum in his very helpful book *The Healing Buddha* (Boulder: Shambhala, 1979), pp.160 and 109 n.21. On p.171 n.11, Birnbaum translates the mantra as: "I honor the Lord Master of Healing, the King of Lapis Lazuli Radiance, Tathāgata, Arhat, Perfectly Enlightened One, saying: To the healing, to the healing, to the supreme healing hail!"

Index